MW00997606

# EAT WELL STAY WELL

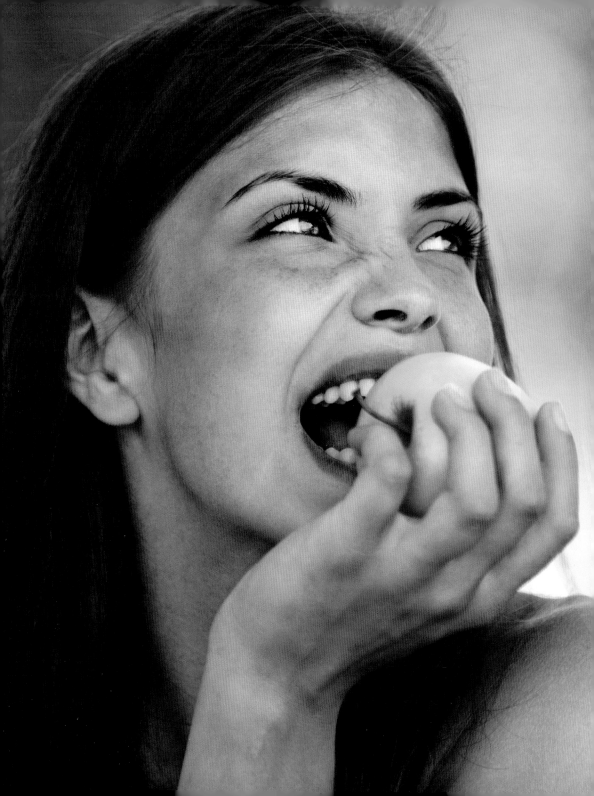

# EAT WELL STAY WELL

## What to eat to beat common ailments

Dr Sarah Brewer

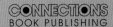

CONNECTIONS
BOOK PUBLISHING

**DEDICATION**

*To my wonderful family for all their support.*

**A CONNECTIONS EDITION**
This edition published in Great Britain in 2013
by Connections Book Publishing Limited
St Chad's House, 148 King's Cross Road
London WC1X 9DH
www.connections-publishing.com

Text copyright © Dr Sarah Brewer 2013
This edition copyright © Eddison Sadd Editions 2013

The right of Dr Sarah Brewer to be identified as the author of this
work has been asserted by her in accordance with the Copyright,
Designs and Patents Act 1988.

All rights reserved. No part of this book may be reproduced, stored
in a retrieval system, or transmitted in any form or by any means without
the prior written permission of the publisher, nor be otherwise circulated
in any form of binding or cover other than that in which it is published and
without a similar condition being imposed on the subsequent purchaser.

British Library Cataloguing-in-Publication data available on request.

ISBN 978-1-85906-371-2

10 9 8 7 6 5 4 3 2

Phototypeset in Benton Gothic, Life and
Weidemann using InDesign on Apple Macintosh
Printed in China

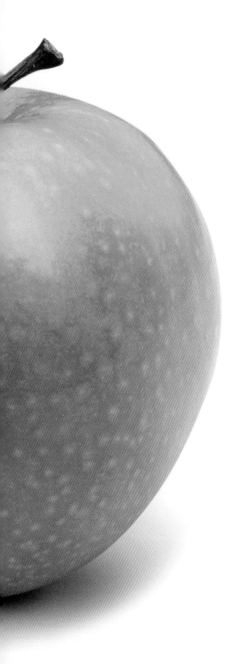

# CONTENTS

# INTRODUCTION

'Let food be your medicine and medicine be your food' is perhaps the most famous saying handed down from Hippocrates of Kos, the Ancient Greek father of modern medicine. Hippocrates firmly believed that a healthy diet was the basis of good health – and, what's more, that ill health could be treated by diet. His admonishment to 'Leave your drugs in the chemist's pot if you can heal the patient with food' had the potential to save a number of lives, given that available treatments of the day included opium, poisonous mushrooms and extensive bloodletting with leeches.

Although he lived around 2,500 years ago, Hippocrates was ahead of his time in recognizing that nutrition is the first line of defence against disease. When your diet is good, 'An apple a day keeps the doctor away.' But when your diet is bad – according to hieroglyphs found in an ancient Egyptian tomb – 'One quarter of what you eat keeps you alive, the other three-quarters provides your doctor's living.' Mark Twain, on the other hand, advised the opposite: 'Eat what you like and let the food fight it out inside.' Unfortunately, 'fighting it out' can result in a number of problems, including indigestion, high cholesterol, diabetes, gout and gallstones, to name but a few.

The food and drink you consume provides all the building blocks needed for your body's growth, repair and maturation. When these building blocks are in optimal supply, your cells can work smoothly. When key nutrients are missing, however, certain metabolic pathways are compromised, cells may not work as efficiently as usual, and premature signs of ageing or failing may occur. Although severe nutritional deficiencies are rare in the Western world, low intakes of certain vitamins and minerals can increase the risk of developing

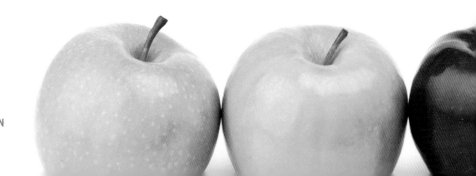

a number of long-term health conditions, including coronary heart disease, stroke, osteoporosis, bone fractures and some cancers.

## About this book

The term 'superfoods' may be a well-used expression these days, but – all hype aside – a number of foods deserve individual attention for their concentrated supply of nutrients with extraordinary nutritional properties. Providing astonishing all-round health benefits, these key foods are reviewed in Part One, along with an overview of the latest scientific research revealing why they have earned their superfood status. These dietary wonders make an invaluable addition to your daily disease-busting arsenal.

Part Two then takes an in-depth look at fifty common health conditions, ranging from asthma and migraines to coronary heart disease and rheumatoid arthritis, exploring which foods are beneficial and, where appropriate, which are best avoided. Organized by ailment – with a handy quick-reference ailment directory, so you can look up what you want, when you want – this section offers clear, straightforward advice that will help you to start taking action right away. Some of my favourite recipes, both nutritious and delicious, are also provided, along with general health tips and advice on supplements that can help, where applicable.

By selecting foods and key nutritional supplements wisely, you will be following the principles of nutritional medicine, which has the potential to prevent, improve and even cure many of the common health problems so prevalent today. Armed with the advice in this book, now you can start eating your way to better health, and staying healthy and happy as you age.

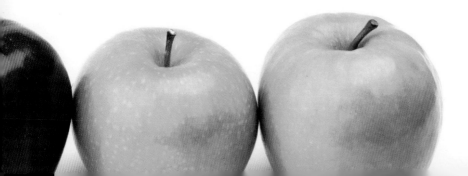

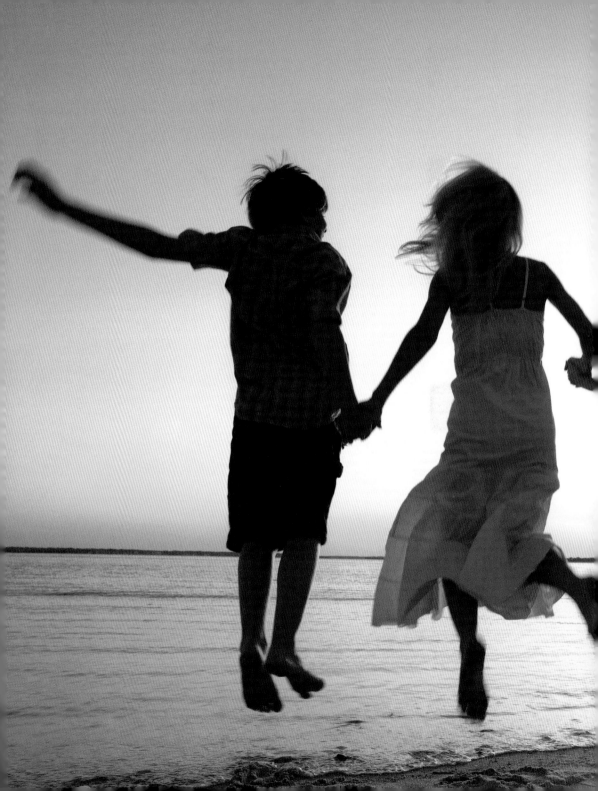

# PART 1
# SUPERFOODS FOR HEALTH

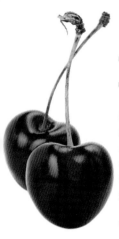

# 1 Cherries

**Cherries range in colour** from yellow and pink to bright red and purple-black. All are rich sources of antioxidant anthocyanins, including chlorogenic acid, quercetin and kaempferol. They're also a good source of vitamin C and potassium.

## DID YOU KNOW?

**Tart cherries** are one of the few rich dietary sources of melatonin – a hormone that helps to promote a good night's sleep.

## The evidence

**Asthma** People with high intakes of quercetin-rich foods, including fresh cherries, have a lower risk of asthma. In addition, young children with asthma who eat a diet rich in vitamin C experience significantly less wheezing than those with low intakes.

**Heart disease** Cherry antioxidants protect blood vessels from oxidative stress and lower levels of monocyte chemoattractant protein-1 (MCP-1), which is involved in furring-up of the arteries (atherosclerosis).

**Arthritis** Cherry juice lowers levels of inflammatory chemicals in the body (such as TNF-alpha) and inhibits inflammatory enzymes (COX-1 and COX-2) – in a similar way to aspirin – to reduce the pain and inflammation associated with arthritis.

**Gout** Eating 250 g (9 oz) black cherries daily, or taking concentrated cherry extracts, can lower uric acid levels enough to prevent gout.

**Insomnia** Montmorency cherry juice improves the quality of sleep by increasing levels of melatonin – the natural hormone responsible for regulating sleep.

**Mood** Cherry juice contains tryptophan, serotonin and melatonin, which can modulate mood and reduce anxiety as well as lowering the stress hormone cortisol.

**Muscle recovery** Montmorency cherry juice has been shown to reduce muscle damage and speed recovery after intensive strength exercise, probably by reducing oxidative damage.

**TRY...**

**Eat fresh or frozen cherries** with yogurt, muesli, fromage frais, fruit salad or any dessert. De-stone and purée to make a rich red coulis to pour over frozen yogurt or other desserts. Add to smoothies, or juice cherries and dilute with apple juice for a refreshing, antioxidant-rich drink. Or dip de-stoned cherries into melted dark chocolate to make a healthy after-dinner treat.

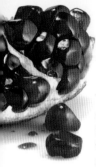

# 2 Pomegranates

**The fleshy arils** (seed casings) of pomegranates contain a ruby-coloured juice that is unusually rich in antioxidants, including a unique group of tannins called punicalagins. Its antioxidant potential is two or three times higher than that of red wine and green tea. Eating just half a pomegranate (100 g/3½ oz) provides as much as 10,500 antioxidant ORAC units (Oxygen Radical Absorbance Capacity).

## The evidence

**Blood pressure**  Pomegranate juice improves arterial dilation by promoting production of nitric oxide, which helps blood vessels relax. Drinking just 50 ml (2 fl oz) pomegranate juice twice a day reduces systolic blood pressure by 5 per cent, by blocking the action of angiotensin-converting enzyme (ACE), an enzyme targeted by many drugs prescribed to lower blood pressure.

**Cholesterol**  Drinking a glass of pomegranate juice per day lowers 'bad' LDL-cholesterol (*see* page 44) and can reverse hardening of the arteries.

**Arterial disease**  According to one study, daily consumption of 240 ml (8 fl oz) pomegranate juice for three months significantly improved blood flow to heart muscle in people with coronary heart disease, compared to a similar group whose condition worsened with a placebo juice. Another study found that daily juice consumption reduced the thickness of the carotid wall lining by up to 35 per cent after one year, while, in a control group not taking the juice, carotid-lining thickness increased by 10 per cent.

**Dental plaque**  Pomegranate fruit extracts have an inhibitory effect on the bacteria causing dental plaque and may help to reduce tooth decay.

### DID YOU KNOW?

**The Kama Sutra** recommends splitting this blushing globe in two and sharing it for increased passion and fertility!

**TRY...**

**Look for pomegranate juice drinks,** or juice your own. Add the seeds to any salad, or try watercress, pear and pomegranate: mix a handful of watercress with a chopped, ripe pear, a few walnuts and the seeds from half a ripe pomegranate; dress with a dash of walnut oil, balsamic vinegar and black pepper. Cutting a fruit in half and picking out the seeds with a blunt pin can be quite therapeutic!

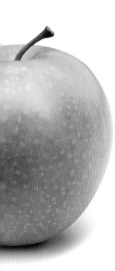

# 3 Apples

**Apples are one of the** richest dietary sources of antioxidant flavonoid polyphenols such as quercetin, which help to reduce inflammation. They also supply pectin, a soluble fibre that blocks the absorption of cholesterol from the intestines, and are good sources of magnesium and boron, essential minerals for health.

## DID YOU KNOW?

**Red apples** provide significantly more antioxidants than green ones. Wash but don't peel your apples – the polyphenols are five times more concentrated in the skin than the flesh. And cloudy apple juice provides more antioxidants than clear juice.

## The evidence

**Longevity** Eating an apple a day can reduce the risk of death from any cause, at any age, by one third, compared with eating less than this. Apples are especially protective against coronary heart disease and stroke – those eating the most apples have a 41 per cent lower risk of thrombotic stroke.

**Cholesterol and weight control**
A study of 160 women who ate an apple a day for a year found that their 'bad' LDL-cholesterol fell by almost a quarter, and their C-reactive protein (an indicator of inflammation in the body) fell by one third. They also each lost around 1.5 kg (3¼ lb) in weight, even though the apples provided additional calories.

**Glucose control** Even sweet apples have a relatively low glycemic index (GI) and help to stabilize blood glucose levels, as the sweetness is mostly provided by the fruit sugar, fructose. Apple flavonoids also protect insulin-producing cells in the pancreas from the progressive damage that occurs in people with impaired glucose tolerance. As a result, a study involving 38,000 women found those eating at least one apple a day were 28 per cent less likely to develop type 2 diabetes than those eating no apples.

**Osteoarthritis** Eating a large (100 g/3½ oz) apple provides the same antioxidant benefits against inflamed joints as 1,500 milligrams of vitamin C.

**TRY...** **Add grated apple** (mix with lemon juice to prevent browning) to salads and coleslaw. Dried apple rings and apple crisps also make a tasty snack. Or make Bircher muesli: soak 1 tbsp rolled oats in 3 tbsp water overnight. To eat, add 1 tbsp lemon juice, 3 tbsp Bio yogurt and 200 g (7 oz) grated apple (don't peel!).

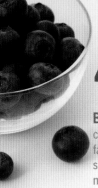

# 4 Berries

**Berries come in a variety** of sizes, colours and flavours. In addition to the familiar types such as blackcurrants, strawberries and blackberries, other more unusual berries such as acai, sea buckthorn and black raspberries can offer key health benefits, too.

## The evidence

**Analgesic** Acai berries are an exceptionally rich source of antioxidants that inhibit enzymes involved in pain and inflammation. Consumption of acai pulp has been shown to have an anti-inflammatory, painkilling effect similar to that of non-steroidal anti-inflammatory drugs (NSAIDs), though the effect is weaker.

**Lung function** Blueberries have one of the highest antioxidant scores of all fruits. Regular consumption has beneficial effects on lung function and may improve asthma, as well as protecting against some of the damage caused by smoking.

**Blood pressure** Bilberries contain antioxidant anthocyanidins such as myrtillin. Regular consumption can lower blood pressure by inhibiting angiotensin-converting enzyme (ACE).

**Colds** Elderberries contain powerful anti-viral substances that can significantly shorten the duration of a cold or flu.

**Muscle stiffness** Blackcurrants are a rich source of anthocyanins, which have been found to reduce shoulder stiffness in typists by increasing peripheral blood flow and reducing muscle fatigue.

**Urinary infections** Cranberries contain substances known as anti-adhesins, which prevent bacteria sticking to cells lining the urinary tract wall. An analysis of ten studies, involving over a thousand people, found that cranberry products were significantly better than placebo in reducing the incidence of recurrent urinary infections in women.

**Dry eyes** Sea buckthorn berries contain an oily blend of omega-3s, -6s, -7s and -9s. Randomized controlled trials have shown that taking 2 g sea buckthorn oil daily for three months reduces redness and burning in people with dry eyes. Sea buckthorn is also used to help improve female intimate dryness.

**Gout** Eating a handful of dark purple-black berries daily can lower uric acid levels enough to prevent an attack of gout.

**TRY...** **Eat fresh or frozen berries.** Add to yogurt, muesli, fromage frais, fruit salads, or any dessert. Purée to make a coulis, or juice berries and dilute with apple juice for a refreshing, antioxidant-rich drink.

### DID YOU KNOW?

**In some parts** of Europe, bilberry extracts are prescribed to reduce excessive bleeding, for patients due to undergo surgery.

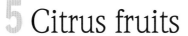

# 5 Citrus fruits

**Citrus fruits such as** lemons, limes, grapefruit and oranges are best known as an excellent source of vitamin C – a single fruit can supply your daily requirement. But they also provide unique citrus bioflavonoids, such as limonene, hesperidin, tangeritin and naringenin, that have anti-inflammatory and anti-cancer properties.

## The evidence

**Asthma** Children who eat citrus fruit on most days in winter are less likely to develop wheeziness than those eating them less than once a week.

**Cholesterol** The pith and membranes of citrus fruit are rich sources of pectin, a soluble fibre that lowers cholesterol levels. Grapefruit also contains bitter naringenin which has cholesterol-lowering properties. Blond and red grapefruit juice can lower LDL-cholesterol (7 per cent for blond, 15 per cent for red), while red grapefruit lowers triglycerides by 17 per cent (5 per cent for blond).

**Blood pressure** Oranges are a rich source of potassium (a single fruit provides 10 per cent of an adult's recommended daily intake), which flushes sodium through the kidneys to reduce fluid retention and lower blood pressure. One study involving the Sweetie (a cross between a grapefruit and pummelo) showed that drinking 500 ml (just under 1 pint) daily significantly lowered blood pressure in people with hypertension, from an average of 142/89 mmHg down to 136/81 mmHg (*see* page 52), within five weeks.

**Cancer** Limonoids and limonene found in citrus fruit have been shown to have anti-cancer properties when tested against cancer cells in the laboratory. A number of studies suggest that people with a high intake of citrus fruit are least likely to develop certain cancers such as of the pancreas and stomach.

**Diabetes** Red 'blood' oranges contain substances which promote insulin secretion and may improve glucose tolerance.

## DID YOU KNOW?

**Unusually for fruits,** oranges also supply thiamin and folate, two important B vitamins. Drinking orange juice with a meal has the additional benefit of helping to boost absorption of iron from the diet.

**TRY...** **Eat at least one citrus fruit** per day, and drink freshly squeezed juice. Using lime juice as a flavouring reduces the need for salt. Or make citrus trout: marinate some trout fillets in the juice and zest of one orange and one lemon; season with freshly ground black pepper and a handful of chopped fresh parsley, and bake or grill for 20 minutes, until cooked through.

**Caution:** *Grapefruit naringenin interferes with the metabolism of some drugs, which can increase the risk of side effects. Check the information sheet supplied with your medication.*

# 6 Grapes

**Black grapes** – traditionally given during convalescence – have long been associated with good health. They contain powerful antioxidant anthocyanidins and phytochemicals (such as resveratrol and pterostilbene) plus potassium, magnesium and trace minerals including boron and copper. Green and pink/red grapes may contain less of the dark red pigments (anthocyanidins), but are still rich in colourless antioxidants (proanthocyanidins) and provide similar health benefits.

## The evidence

**Asthma** Children who eat a lot of grapes are least likely to develop wheezing or rhinitis.

**Blood pressure** Grape flavonoids can lower blood pressure through a combination of relaxing smooth muscle in arterial linings, having a blood-thinning action, and by blocking the activity of an enzyme (ACE) that is also targeted by antihypertensive drugs. In one study, drinking around 300 ml (half a pint) of Concord red grape juice daily was found to reduce blood pressure by an average of 7.2/6.2 mmHg after eight weeks.

**Circulation** Antioxidant flavonoids found in grapeseed are similar to those found in grape juice and wine. They have a beneficial effect on the circulation, by inhibiting oxidation of 'bad' LDL-cholesterol and the formation of unwanted blood clots, and relaxing blood vessel linings. They also appear to strengthen fragile capillaries and protect cell structures from damaging oxidation reactions. Grapeseed extracts are available in tablet form as a food supplement.

**Cancer** Grapes are a source of substances such as ellagic acid, piceatannol and resveratrol, which have been shown to have anti-cancer properties in laboratory tests.

> ### DID YOU KNOW?
>
> **Although grape seeds** constitute less than 5 per cent of the weight of a grape, they contain two-thirds of their flavonoid content.

**TRY...**

**Eat a handful of grapes** – fresh or dried (raisins, currants, sultanas) – as a healthy snack, or drink a glass of red grape juice, either on its own or mixed with other juices. Or use grape juice in home-made jellies or fresh fruit salads: chop black seedless grapes, orange segments, ripe pears, melons and bananas; half cover with red or green grape juice and serve.

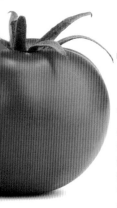

# 7 Tomatoes

**Tomatoes contain** a red pigment called lycopene that protects the plant from sunburn. It is a powerful antioxidant that, among other benefits, also helps to protect our skin from sun exposure. When cooked, tomatoes release five times more lycopene than is available in their raw state. Tomato ketchup and tomato purée (which are concentrated) are therefore rich dietary sources.

## The evidence

**Heart disease** Lycopene reduces oxidation of the 'bad' LDL-cholesterol associated with atherosclerosis (hardening and narrowing of the arteries). It also protects against abnormal blood clots, and improves arterial flexibility by 50 per cent. People who regularly eat tomatoes and tomato products are at least a third less likely to develop coronary heart disease than those who eat them infrequently.

**Cancer** Lycopene is a potent antioxidant, and a single serving of tomatoes can reduce DNA oxidative damage by as much as 50 per cent within 24 hours. People with the highest tomato intakes, and blood lycopene levels, are least likely to develop cancers of the mouth, oesophagus, stomach,

**DID YOU KNOW?**

**As lycopene** is fat-soluble, drizzling your margherita pizza with olive oil increases your dietary absorption of lycopene as much as threefold.

lung, colon, rectum, cervix and prostate gland. Consuming more than 10 servings of tomato products per week reduces the risk of prostate cancer by a third, compared with men eating less than 1.5 servings per week. Women with the highest lycopene levels are also five times less likely to have an abnormal cervical smear than women with very low lycopene levels.

**AMD** Those with low lycopene intakes have more than double the risk of developing age-related macular degeneration (*see* page 72) than those with high intakes.

**Asthma** Women with a high intake of tomatoes are 15 per cent less likely to have asthma than those with very low intakes. Lycopene can also protect against exercise-induced asthma.

**Skin** Lycopene is depleted in skin exposed to ultraviolet light, suggesting that it also plays a role in protecting the skin from sun damage.

**TRY...** **Drink tomato juice,** or make tomato-based soups, stews and sauces: arrange fresh, halved tomatoes on a tray, drizzle with olive oil, oregano and crushed garlic and bake for 30 minutes, then whizz in a blender to make a fresh sauce for pasta. Or serve roast tomatoes with fish and meats.

# 8 Beetroot

**These dark red** root vegetables have a sweet, earthy flavour and are a rich source of antioxidant phytochemicals. Unlike in most other dark-purple plants, the deep beetroot colour is not due to anthocyanin pigments but to the presence of a red pigment known as betanin. Betanin is water-soluble, and high intakes can cause a temporary, harmless red discolouration of urine (beeturia).

## The evidence

**Blood pressure** Beetroot is a rich source of magnesium, potassium and natural nitrates, all of which have a blood-pressure-lowering action. Nitrates are broken down to form nitrites by bacteria that live on the surface of your tongue. When you swallow the resulting nitrite-rich saliva, the nitrites are absorbed via the stomach into your circulation. Within blood vessels, nitrites form nitric oxide, which has a powerful relaxing effect on small muscles in blood vessel linings. This causes the vessels to dilate, so that blood pressure falls. Drinking just 70 ml (2½ fl oz) beetroot juice can reduce resting blood pressure by 2 per cent, while drinking 500 ml (almost a pint) can significantly lower blood pressure within an hour, with the effect lasting up to 24 hours.

**Homocysteine** Betaine helps to lower blood levels of homocysteine, a harmful amino acid that is linked with hardening and furring up of the arteries.

**Memory** Beetroot improves blood flow to the brain, thereby improving mental performance. Researchers recently suggested that a daily glass of beetroot juice might reduce the onset of dementia among older adults.

**Exercise performance** Beetroot makes muscles more efficient at burning fuel, to reduce the oxygen cost of walking and running. Some studies have found that (in moderately trained subjects; performance does not appear to be enhanced in highly trained athletes) ingesting beetroot juice 3 hours before exercise can shave 1–2 per cent off the time taken to cycle trial distances of between 4 km and 16 km (2½–10 miles).

## DID YOU KNOW?

**200 g (7 oz) cooked beetroot** contains a similar level of blood-vessel-dilating nitrates to 500 ml (just under 1 pint) beetroot juice.

**TRY...**

**Drink beetroot juice,** or eat cooked beetroot plain, pickled with balsamic vinegar, or mixed with spring onions, chickpeas or beans as a salad. Beetroot crisps also make a healthy snack. Or make beetroot and butterbean hummus: blend 250 g (9 oz) cooked beetroot with a tin of drained butterbeans, 1 clove garlic, a small bunch of fresh chives and 3 tbsp extra virgin olive oil; season with black pepper and vinegar to taste (for more beetroot recipes, visit www.lovebeetroot.co.uk).

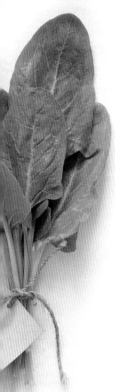

# 9 Spinach

**Popeye's favourite** energizing food, spinach is one of the richest sources of folate, a vitamin involved in a wide number of metabolic reactions. Deficiency quickly leads to tiredness, lack of energy and, if not corrected, a form of anaemia. Spinach also supplies good amounts of antioxidant carotenoids plus vitamins C and E, as well as calcium and iron.

## The evidence

**AMD** Spinach is one of the richest dietary sources of the carotenoids lutein and zeaxanthin, which help to protect against age-related macular degeneration (*see* page 72). A typical serving of cooked spinach provides 20 mg lutein, compared with 2 mg for broccoli.

**Cancer** Due to its role in chromosome replication during cell division, dietary folate obtained from regular consumption of spinach may protect against the development of certain cancers, including of the cervix, oesophagus, mouth, bowel, lung and breast – especially in smokers.

**Bones** Spinach is an excellent source of calcium, needed for strong bones and teeth, as well as for muscle contraction and nerve conduction.

DID YOU **KNOW?**

**The iron** in spinach is less well absorbed than haem iron (found in meat), but the high amount of vitamin C in green leafy vegetables helps to keep the inorganic form of iron in the ferrous state for maximum absorption.

**Fatigue** In a study of sixty people with chronic fatigue syndrome, half had low levels of folic acid. Spinach helps make muscles more efficient at burning fuel, to reduce the oxygen cost of walking and running.

**Blood pressure** Spinach is rich in nitrates and at least four peptides with the ability to inhibit angiotensin-converting enzyme (ACE) and lower blood pressure. The Dietary Approaches to Stop Hypertension (DASH) trials showed that you can significantly reduce your blood pressure within eight weeks by eating more fruit and veg, including spinach.

**Asthma** Those with the highest intake of green leafy vegetables are 18 per cent less likely to have asthma than those with very low intakes.

**Memory** Green leafy vegetables, including spinach, appear to help slow age-related mental decline.

**TRY...** **Eat it raw or lightly steamed** (wilted), and use as an accompaniment to any meal. Baby leaves are great in salads. Add spinach leaves when juicing fruit and vegetables – you won't taste the difference. Or try a spinach omelette: sauté some sliced spring onions, garlic, spinach and fresh herbs; add 2 whisked eggs, season with freshly ground black pepper and cook until set.

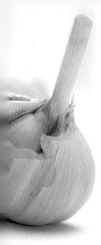

# 10 Garlic

**Garlic was used by** the Ancient Egyptians to treat a variety of conditions ranging from heart disease and worms to cancer. Over 3,000 years later, modern medicine has confirmed its beneficial effects in these areas – and more.

## DID YOU KNOW?

**Black garlic** – produced by fermenting bulbs under controlled conditions – offers all the health benefits, without the strong odour. Its savoury-sweet flavour is reminiscent of molasses and balsamic with garlic undertones.

## The evidence

**Cholesterol** Allicin (the key beneficial compound in garlic, released when it is cut or crushed) reduces cholesterol production in the liver and also prevents cells from taking up cholesterol. Taking garlic tablets can lower harmful LDL-cholesterol by up to 12 per cent and triglycerides by up to 27 per cent.

**Circulation** Garlic boosts blood flow through small arteries by almost 50 per cent. This can improve symptoms associated with poor circulation, such as Raynaud's disease and chilblains.

**Blood thinning** Garlic reduces formation of unwanted blood clots. Some of its ingredients are as potent as aspirin, and may help to reduce the risk of heart attack and some forms of stroke.

**Allergies** Anecdotal evidence suggests that black-garlic extract may reduce symptoms of rhinitis and watering eyes.

**Blood pressure** Sulphur compounds formed from the breakdown of allicin relax blood vessels to lower blood pressure. Trials suggests that garlic extracts reduce BP by an average of 16.3/9.3 mmHg in people with hypertension.

**Cancer** Garlic suppresses the formation of cancer-causing substances in the intestines. Studies suggest that people consuming more than 28.8 g (1 oz) per week are almost a third less likely to develop colorectal cancer, and half less likely to develop stomach cancer, as those consuming less than 3.5 g (⅛ oz) a week.

**Obesity** Black-garlic extract inhibits fat accumulation in fat cells, and may play a supportive role in weight loss. It may also reduce fat accumulation in liver cells.

**Infections** According to one study, taking garlic supplements for twelve weeks reduces the chance of developing a cold and, if one occurs, shortens its duration.

**TRY...**

**Use garlic in all savoury dishes** – add towards the end of cooking for maximum effect. Or make Greek almond and garlic relish: blend together 4 large cloves garlic, 150 ml (¼ pint) extra virgin olive oil, 1 slice bread, 30 ml (1 fl oz) white wine vinegar and 100 g (3½ oz) ground almonds; season with black pepper.

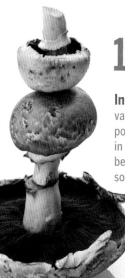

# 11 Mushrooms

**In addition to** the more familiar varieties such as white, chestnut and porcini, medicinal mushrooms – revered in Asia for over 3,000 years – are becoming increasingly available. While some are sold fresh, such as shiitake, many are only available dried (such as maitake) or in tablet form (reishi). Only use exotic 'wild' mushrooms from a trusted source, as some varieties are poisonous.

## The evidence

**Cholesterol** Reishi extracts have been shown to significantly decrease blood cholesterol, LDL-cholesterol and triglycerides; healthy volunteers taking reishi for four weeks showed a trend towards lower blood cholesterol and increased antioxidant activity.

**Blood pressure** People with a high intake of mushrooms have a blood pressure around 5 mmHg lower than those who eat few. Some edible mushrooms (such as Tricholoma giganteum, common in Japan and Australia, reishi and maitake) lower BP by blocking the action of angiotensin-converting enzyme (ACE) in a similar way to some antihypertensive drugs.

## DID YOU KNOW?

**Bought wild-mushroom soup** can contain less than 1 per cent wild mushrooms, with factory-produced button mushrooms making up the bulk. Make your own instead!

**Immunity** Medicinal mushrooms such as Tricholoma giganteum, reishi, maitake, Phellinus linteus and shiitake contain immune-modulating proteoglycans, which are used in Japan to boost the body's defences against cancer, viral and fungal infections. Reishi extracts are said to 'dramatically' decrease pain associated with shingles and post-herpetic neuralgia.

**Prostate** Reishi has anti-androgen activity. A study involving eighty-eight men with lower urinary tract symptoms related to benign prostate enlargement found it improved the International Prostate Symptoms Score without affecting testosterone levels.

**Weight** Substituting white button mushrooms for beef in dishes such as lasagne and chilli can halve the calorie content of the meal without reducing palatability or satisfaction, as they provide the same volume and filling power. Doing this once a week for a year would help you lose 5 lb (2.3 kg) in weight.

## TRY...

**Slice mushrooms raw into salads,** sauté in olive oil with garlic, parboil in bouillon, or bake in the oven, stuffed with mashed butternut squash and parsley. Or make creamy mushroom toasties: sauté thin slices of red onion with garlic, fresh herbs (thyme, parsley) and a handful of mushrooms until soft; bind with a little low-fat crème fraîche, season with black pepper and serve on rye toast. Take reishi or maitake as supplements.

# 12 Soybeans

**Soybeans contain** isoflavones, a class of plant hormones. When eaten, these are broken down by bacteria in your large intestine to release the active forms genistein and daidzein, which have an oestrogen-like action in the body. Although far weaker than human oestrogen, they still provide a significant hormone boost.

## The evidence

**Menopause** Several studies show that soy isoflavones can reduce menopausal hot flushes and night sweats by at least a third. This may explain why less than 25 per cent of women following an Asian diet complain of hot flushes, compared with 85 per cent of Western women.

**Pre-menstrual syndrome** Isoflavone supplements can reduce symptoms of headache, breast tenderness, cramps and swelling, compared with placebo.

### DID YOU KNOW?

**In Asia,** where soy is a dietary staple, isoflavone intakes average 50–100 mg per day, compared with typical Western intakes of just 2–5 mg daily.

**Osteoporosis** An analysis of ten studies found significant increases in spine bone mineral density in those consuming soy isoflavones, compared with those with low intakes.

**Heart disease** Soy isoflavones interact with oestrogen receptors within the circulation, helping to dilate coronary arteries, reduce arterial stiffness, lower blood pressure, and reduce LDL-cholesterol, blood stickiness and platelet clumping. Consuming 40 g (1½ oz) soybean protein per day can reduce blood pressure by at least 7/5 mmHg within twelve weeks.

**Memory** Consuming a high soy diet has been found to improve memory and frontal-lobe function in young healthy students (both male and female), men and postmenopausal women.

**Prostate cancer** An analysis of twenty-four trials found that non-fermented soy products reduced the relative risk of developing prostate cancer by 30 per cent, and taking isoflavone supplements reduced the risk by 12 per cent.

**Breast cancer** A study of 21,852 Japanese women found that those with the highest intake of isoflavones were 54 per cent less likely to develop breast cancer, even after adjusting for other factors.

**TRY...** **Use soybeans in soups, stews and stir-fries,** select soybean products such as tofu and low-salt soy sauce, or add soybean protein powder to shakes. Or enjoy in apple muesli: place a handful of porridge oats in a bowl, scatter with raisins, walnuts and a sprinkle of cinnamon, add soy milk to cover, mix and soak in the fridge overnight. Before serving, stir through 1 grated apple and, if desired, some unsweetened apple juice.

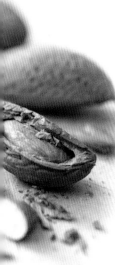

# 13 Nuts

## Nuts are a rich source of

antioxidants, vitamins, minerals and monounsaturated and omega-3 oils, both of which have beneficial effects in the body. Yet, in a study examining dietary intakes across ten European countries, only 4.4 per cent of just under 37,000 people reported eating tree nuts over the previous 24 hours, and only 2.3 per cent recalled eating peanuts.

## The evidence

**Cholesterol** Nuts reduce the absorption of cholesterol, due to their soluble fibre and phytosterol content. Their flavanol antioxidants also prevent oxidation of LDL-cholesterol so it is more readily carried back to the liver for processing. As a result, eating a handful of nuts a day lowers your 'bad' LDL-cholesterol and increases your 'good' HDL-cholesterol enough to reduce your risk of a heart attack or stroke by at least 20 per cent.

**Cancer** Brazil nuts are the richest dietary source of selenium, needed for the production of powerful antioxidant enzymes. The minimum daily intake required for optimum anti-cancer protection is 75–125 mcg per day – supplied by eating two to three Brazils.

## DID YOU KNOW?

**Tree nuts include** almonds, Brazils, cashews, hazelnuts, macadamias, pecans, pistachios and walnuts. Peanuts, or groundnuts, are actually legumes (beans).

**Weight** Although nuts are high in calories, their consumption does not cause a net gain in body weight when eaten as a replacement food. Nuts have a high protein content, which curbs appetite. Studies show that those who eat nuts regularly tend to have a lower body mass index (BMI) than those who eat few, despite an increase in total fat consumed.

**Heart disease** Monounsaturated and omega-3 essential fatty acids help to protect against heart disease. A recent study involving over 13,000 adults showed that regular nut consumption was associated with a lower prevalence of four risk factors for heart disease: blood pressure, cholesterol, weight and high-fasting glucose.

**Hormone balance** Nuts are a good source of oestrogen-like phytochemicals, especially almonds, cashews, hazelnuts, peanuts, walnuts and nut oils. Eating nuts is especially beneficial around the time of the menopause.

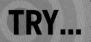

**TRY...** **Add nuts to cereals,** desserts, yogurts, salads and home-made breads. Use nut oils in salad dressings, and drink nut milk (available in health food stores). Or toast nuts for a healthy snack: warm a pan over a medium heat, pour in a handful of unsalted mixed shelled nuts, and toast gently for a few seconds, shaking the pan as they turn golden (don't burn!). Turn out into a shallow dish and leave to cool.

# 14 Olive oil

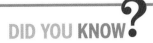

**DID YOU KNOW?**

- 1 tbsp olive oil contains 15 g (½ oz) total fat, of which only 2 g is saturated fat.
- 1 tbsp butter contains 12 g (²/₅ oz) total fat, of which 8 g is saturated fat.

**Olive oil is an essential** part of the ultra-healthy Mediterranean diet. Its principal component – monounsaturated oleic acid – reduces absorption of cholesterol and is processed in the body to lower total and 'bad' LDL-cholesterol without modifying the 'good' HDL-cholesterol. It also reduces abnormal blood clotting and has beneficial effects on glucose control.

## The evidence

**Blood pressure** In one study, 80 per cent of people on medication for high blood pressure were able to discontinue their medication after using 30–40 g (1–1½ oz) olive oil for cooking every day for six months. Those using sunflower oil continued to need antihypertensive treatment.

**Stroke** The blood-pressure-lowering effect of olive oil can reduce your risk of a stroke by up to 70 per cent.

**Cholesterol balance** Olive oil contains plant sterols that help to block the absorption of cholesterol in the gut. It's also processed in the liver to reduce production of harmful LDL-cholesterol and to lower blood levels of triglycerides (another type of fat). These effects are greatest with virgin and extra virgin olive oils, compared with pure olive oil (which is a blend).

**Glucose control** Oleic acid improves insulin sensitivity. Replacing some dietary carbohydrate with 10–40 g (¼–1½ oz) olive oil per day can help people with type 2 diabetes, and could potentially prevent over 90 per cent of cases.

**Heart disease** A diet rich in olive oil (34 per cent total fat, with 21 per cent as monounsaturated fatty acid and only 7 per cent as saturated fat) can reduce your risk of a heart attack by 25 per cent.

**TRY...**

**Use pure olive oil** for frying and roasting (it remains stable at elevated temperatures), and reserve extra virgin and virgin olive oils for gentle braising, drizzling over foods and for salads. For a herby dressing, place 60 ml (2 fl oz) extra virgin olive oil, 3 tsp red wine vinegar, 1 clove crushed garlic, a handful of chopped fresh herbs and a twist of ground black pepper in a small jar with screw-top lid. Cover, shake jar to emulsify, then pour over your salad.

# 15 Chocolate

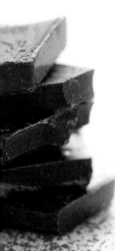

**Dark-chocolate cocoa solids** contain more antioxidant flavonoids than just about any other food (dark chocolate has five times more antioxidant activity than the same weight of blueberries, for example). While some flavonoids contain just one unit (monomers), dark chocolate is especially rich in those containing two, three or more units (oligomers), which have the greatest health benefits.

## The evidence

**Heart disease** Dark chocolate has been shown to increase insulin sensitivity and 'good' HDL-cholesterol, and to decrease blood pressure and 'bad' LDL-cholesterol, while reducing unwanted blood-cell clumping and inflammation. Researchers have discovered that eating 45 g (1½ oz) dark chocolate per day significantly increases blood flow through the coronary arteries, as it prevents harmful LDL-cholesterol from becoming oxidized and taken up into artery walls.

**Blood pressure** Research published in the *British Medical Journal* shows that eating 100 g (3½ oz) dark chocolate per day can reduce blood pressure by an average of 5.1/1.8 mmHg, which is enough to reduce the risk of a heart attack or stroke by 21 per cent. In another study, older males drinking high quantities of cocoa were found to have a BP 3.7/2.1 mmHg lower than in those

> ### DID YOU KNOW?
>
> **According to** the *New England Journal of Medicine*, countries with the highest chocolate consumption per head of population produce the most Nobel Prize winners.

drinking very little – and they were half as likely to die of cardiovascular (or any other illness) during a fifteen-year follow-up.

**Asthma** Dark chocolate contains theobromine, a methylxanthine used as a drug to help dilate the airways. It is also a more effective cough-suppressant than codeine – a component of over-the-counter cough medicines. An edible spacer device (an add-on device for inhalers), made from chocolate, has also been found to improve the bronchodilator effect of reliever inhalers in children!

**TRY...** **Select dark chocolate** containing at least 72 per cent cocoa solids, and eat after a meal when you're less likely to over-indulge. For an after-dinner treat, blend 200 g (7 oz) silken tofu (soft) with the juice and zest of one orange; spoon bite-sized dollops onto a baking sheet and freeze, then dip the frozen balls into melted dark chocolate and refreeze. **Note:** 100 g (3½ oz) dark chocolate contains 510 kcals, so limit the amount you eat if you're watching your weight.

# 16 Red wine

**Wine contains** a rich selection of antioxidants (including flavonoids, flavonols, catechins, anthocyanins, procyanidins and soluble tannins), derived from the juice and skins of grapes. Red wine contains higher amounts than white, as it is left in contact with grape-skin pigments for longer.

## The evidence

**Cholesterol** Red wine antioxidants inhibit the uptake and oxidation of cholesterol. A moderate intake (250 ml/8½ fl oz red wine daily) decreases total and 'bad 'LDL-cholesterol, while increasing circulating levels of 'good' HDL-cholesterol.

**Blood pressure** Alcohol has a relaxing effect, which lowers stress and promotes dilation of arteries. A study in which subjects drank 250 ml (8½ fl oz) red wine per night for fifteen days found that blood pressure decreased by 7 mmHg. Higher intakes, however, are associated with a rise in blood pressure.

**Blood clotting** Red wine antioxidants have a blood-thinning action, helping to prevent the formation of unwanted blood clots – partly by reducing levels of the blood-clotting factor fibrinogen, and partly by reducing the stickiness of circulating cell fragments (platelets).

**Heart disease** People who consume one to two drinks per day have up to a 50 per cent reduction in calcification of the coronary arteries, compared with non-drinkers. Pooled data from thirty-four studies, involving over a million people, shows the risk of coronary heart disease decreased with intakes of up to four drinks per day in men, and two drinks per day in women. However, at higher intakes this protection is lost due to higher blood pressure and the development of abnormal heart rhythms.

**Cancer** Regular, moderate wine consumption (one to two glasses a day) is associated with a lower risk of certain types of cancer, including colon, basal cell, ovarian, and prostate carcinoma. Conversely, however, each unit of alcohol increases the risk of breast cancer.

## DID YOU KNOW?

**Red wines** made from the Argentinian Malbec grape, the Italian Sangiovese grape, and the Madiran Tannat grape (France) contain the highest levels of beneficial antioxidants.

**TRY...**

**Drink 1 small glass** (125 ml/4 fl oz) of red wine daily (if drinking more than this, aim to have two or more alcohol-free days per week). Or make pears in red wine: peel and halve some firm pears, cover with red wine, add a sprinkle of cinnamon and the juice and zest of an orange; simmer, turning frequently, until pears are tender, then remove pears and boil liquor to reduce by half. Sweeten with stevia (a natural sweetener) to your taste, then pour over the pears. Serve hot or chilled.

# 17 Tea

**Green, white, black,** oolong and pu-erh teas are all made from the young leaves of the same shrub, *Camellia sinensis*. Tea leaves contain high levels (up to 30 per cent by weight) of flavonoid catechins, making this refreshing drink a rich source of antioxidants. Tea also contains the trace element manganese, and is one of the few dietary sources of fluoride.

## The evidence

**Heart disease** Drinking tea has beneficial effects on blood lipids, blood pressure and blood stickiness, and can decrease the risk of coronary heart disease and stroke. Researchers have suggested that people who drink at least four cups of tea a day are up to half as likely to have a heart attack as non-tea drinkers, and 21 per cent less likely to have a stroke.

**Diabetes** People who drink four or more cups of tea per day are 27 per cent less likely to develop type 2 diabetes than those drinking none. In one study, those with type 2 diabetes who drank 1500 ml (almost 3 pints) oolong tea daily for thirty days reduced their blood glucose levels by 30 per cent, compared with a similar period when drinking water.

## DID YOU KNOW?

**If you're watching your** caffeine intake, choose your tea carefully: white tea contains around 15 mg caffeine per cup, compared to 20 mg for green tea and 40 mg for black tea.

**Cancer** Analysis of results from four studies suggests that women with the highest intake of tea are 22 per cent less likely to develop breast cancer.

**Asthma** Tea contains substances (caffeine, theobromine and theophylline) that help to dilate the airways. Drinking tea two or three times a day can reduce the risk of asthma by 28 per cent.

**Stress** Tea contains theanine, an amino acid that helps to reduce stress and promote relaxation.

**Weight loss** Green tea boosts the rate at which the body burns calories by as much as 40 per cent over a 24-hour period. It may also block the activity of intestinal enzymes needed to digest dietary fat, so that less fat is absorbed. Several trials suggest that adding green tea extracts to a weight loss regime helps to improve fat loss; a study of sixty obese adults showed a loss of 11 kg/24 lb over three months.

**TRY...** **Drink green, black or white tea regularly,** three to five times a day. Use leftover cold tea to soak dried fruit, as a basis for sauces, soups or stews, or to make ice cream. Or try green tea compote: pour hot green tea over chopped semi-dried apricots, prunes, dates, figs and raisins and leave to steep until cold. Serve with low-fat fromage frais or bio yogurt, scattered with pistachio nuts.

# 18 Spices

**Spices contain** a potent mix of unique chemicals that contribute to their pungency. While only used in small amounts, they often provide more antioxidants than a serving of fruit or vegetables: just 1 g of black pepper, for example, has a similar antioxidant score to 100 g (3½ oz) of tomatoes.

## The evidence

**Pain** Chilli peppers contain capsaicin, which blocks the transmission of pain messages in nerves, as well as triggering the release of endorphins – the brain's own morphine-like painkillers. Other spices with analgesic properties include star anise, cloves, cumin, fennel, ginger, mustard and turmeric.

**Circulation** Capsaicin in chilli peppers can lower blood pressure by dilating blood vessels. Cinnamon, fenugreek and ginger have all been found to lower triglycerides, total and LDL-cholesterol.

**Arthritis** Turmeric and ginger contain curcumin, which has a powerful anti-inflammatory action equivalent to that of some prescribed corticosteroid drugs, to reduce cartilage destruction in osteoarthritis.

## DID YOU KNOW?

**Cloves have the** highest antioxidant score of all the spices (3,144 units per gram), followed by cinnamon (2,675), turmeric (1,592), nutmeg (1,572) and cumin (768).

**Asthma** Curcumin is used in Ayurvedic and Chinese medicine to treat respiratory diseases such as asthma. It appears to relax smooth muscles to reduce bronchospasm, cough and mucus production.

**Diabetes** Cinnamon is believed to promote the secretion of insulin from pancreatic beta-cells. In people with type 2 diabetes, cinnamon extracts were shown to improve blood glucose levels by 10–29 per cent. Preliminary research suggests ginger may reduce diabetes-related kidney damage, while fenugreek was found to halve the amount of glucose in urine.

**Bowel conditions** Turmeric extracts can halve the severity of irritable bowel symptoms. In people with ulcerative colitis, adding turmeric extracts to their usual medication regime significantly reduced the chance of relapse.

**Nausea** Ginger is an effective treatment for post-operative nausea and vomiting, motion sickness and nausea in pregnancy.

**TRY...** **Add spices to curries, soups, stews,** and use turmeric to colour rice dishes and desserts. Drink turmeric or ginger tea, or dry ginger ale. Or make spicy baked apples: wash and core cooking apples and stand in a small baking dish. Stud each with 4 cloves, fill the apple centres with raisins, a knob of butter and a dash of cinnamon. Sweeten some hot ginger tea with stevia and pour over the apples to a depth of around 3 mm. Bake for 45 minutes until soft.

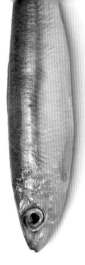

# 19 Oily fish

**Oily fish are a rich source of** long-chain omega-3 fatty acids, especially EPA and DHA. These are converted in the body into substances that regulate immune reactions and reduce inflammation. (Non-fish sources of omega-3s include blue-green algae, walnuts, flaxseed and hemp oils, and vegetarian supplements containing DHA from algae are available.)

## The evidence

**Heart disease** Omega-3 fish oils have a beneficial effect on blood pressure, blood stickiness and blood fat levels. They may also protect against certain abnormal heart rhythms, especially in heart muscle receiving a poor blood supply. Even a modest increase in dietary intakes of oily fish can reduce your chance of a heart attack.

**Stroke** People who eat oily fish on a weekly basis regularly are 12 per cent less likely to die from a stroke than those who don't, with possible additional reductions of 2 per cent per serving per week, if you eat more.

**AMD** Omega-3 fish oils may protect against progression of age-related macular degeneration.

**DID YOU KNOW?**

**Oily fish include:** anchovies (unsalted), bloater, cacha, carp, eel, herring, hilsa, jack fish, katla, kipper, mackerel, orange roughy, pangas, pilchards, salmon, sardines, sprats, swordfish, trout, tuna (fresh, but not tinned), whitebait.

**Inflammatory disease** Eating fish two or three times a week reduces the risk of asthma, inflammatory bowel disease, rheumatoid arthritis and psoriasis. Their analgesic effect is similar to non-steroidal anti-inflammatory drugs in helping to reduce joint pain and swelling.

**Brain health** Omega-3 fish oils play an important structural role within brain-cell membranes, improving their fluidity so that messages are passed on more rapidly from one cell to another. They also have a beneficial effect against depression.

**Cancer** Fish oils may reduce the risk of cancer by interfering with the growth of tumour cells and reversing the weight loss that can occur in people with cancer. A number of trials suggest that each additional 100 g (3½ oz) of fish you consume per week lowers the risk of bowel cancer by around 3 per cent.

**TRY...** **Eat fish as fresh as possible,** and preferably raw (sushi, sashimi), steamed, grilled or baked until just cooked. Or make nutty oatmeal herrings: dip a herring fillet in milk, then roll in a mixture of coarse oatmeal, chopped pecans and crushed black pepper. Fry in olive oil, over gentle heat, until cooked; sprinkle with lemon juice and serve on a bed of watercress.

# 20 Yogurt

**Live yogurt is a** fermented milk product containing beneficial bacteria. These produce lactic acid and are often referred to as 'probiotics'. Because these are acid tolerant, a significant number survive through the stomach to reach the large intestine, where they discourage the growth of gas-forming bacteria, stimulate immunity, and aid digestion.

## The evidence

**Blood pressure** Lactic-acid bacteria can reduce hypertension by blocking angiotensin-converting enzyme (ACE) – which is also targeted by many hypertension drugs. The mineral content of dairy foods such as yogurt has also been shown to reduce the risk of hypertension and stroke.

**Allergies** Lactic-acid bacteria may reduce the development of allergic conditions such as asthma and eczema by stimulating the immune system to produce antibodies rather than triggering an allergic response. Studies found that the offspring of women who took probiotics during pregnancy were less likely to develop eczema, at least during their early years.

**Irritable bowel syndrome** A large analysis of fourteen trials suggests that replenishing the bowel population of lactic-acid-producing bacteria can improve IBS symptoms when used alone or in combination with standard anti-spasm medications.

**Diarrhoea** Some yogurt bacteria inhibit the growth of harmful bacteria that cause gastroenteritis, such as *Salmonella*, *Shigella* and *Clostridium*. They can also reduce diarrhoea caused by taking some antibiotics.

**Colds** Vitamins, minerals and probiotics work together to bolster immunity. Studies show that those taking probiotics plus multivitamins and minerals were less likely to develop cold and flu symptoms than those taking multivitamins alone, the severity of symptoms was reduced, and the number of days with fever more than halved. All immune cells showed increased activity.

**Thrush** Lactic-acid-producing bacteria naturally found in the gut are believed to inhibit the growth of yeasts responsible for vaginal Candida infections (thrush). Taking both probiotics and the anti-fungal drug fluconazole can significantly improve treatment response, with less discharge and a lower presence of yeasts.

**TRY...** **Eat live bio yogurt with** breakfast cereals, or with chopped fruit as a dessert. Stir into soups and sauces, and use in salad dressings and smoothies. Or make berry crunch: top a handful of fresh berries with low-fat vanilla bio yogurt, scatter with granola and enjoy!

## DID YOU KNOW?

**Nobel Prize winner**
Ilya Mechnikov believed live yogurt, containing *L. bulgaricus*, contributed to the long lifespan of Bulgarian peasants.

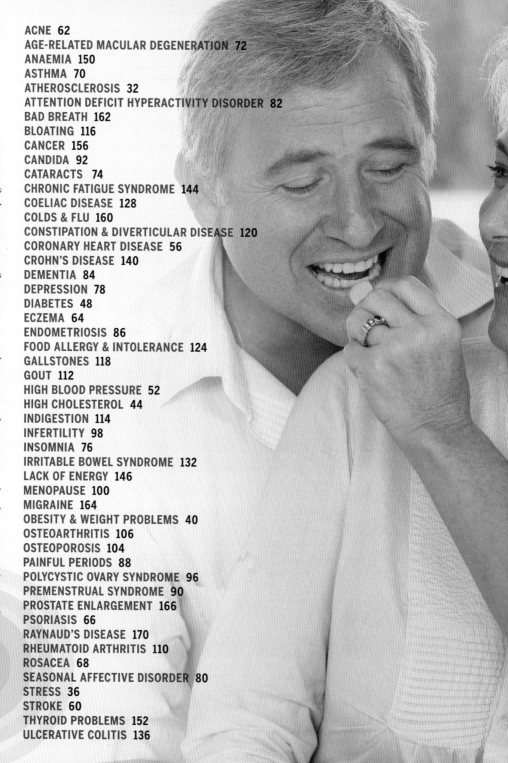

## QUICK-REFERENCE AILMENT DIRECTORY

*For quick reference to a specific ailment, refer to this alphabetical listing to check the page number:*

WHAT TO EAT – AND WHAT TO AVOID – TO HELP ALLEVIATE AND PREVENT FIFTY COMMON AILMENTS

**PART 2**
# EAT TO BEAT...

# Atherosclerosis

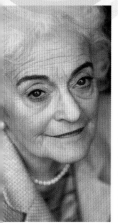

**Atherosclerosis is the hardening** and furring-up of the arteries. This starts early in life as an accumulation of fatty streaks along major artery walls; by the age of fifty, most people are affected. But foods rich in antioxidants, folic acid and vitamins $B_6$ and $B_{12}$ can help.

Atherosclerosis is the body's response to wear-and-tear damage in artery walls. This damage can result from uncontrolled high blood pressure, raised cholesterol levels, diabetes, smoking or eating a poor diet – especially one that's high in fat and low in antioxidants. Once damage occurs, small circulating cell fragments (platelets) form a tiny clot to stimulate healing. If excessive damage continues, low-grade inflammation attracts scavenger cells which, if laden with oxidized cholesterol (scavenged from the circulation), become trapped to form fatty deposits.

Over time, these build up to form raised plaques (atheroma) that bulge into the space inside the artery, causing narrowing. Inflammation also causes the underlying artery wall to degenerate, so it becomes fibrous and more stiff. Loss of elasticity means that blood-pressure surges, which occur with each heartbeat, are not evened out. If atherosclerosis is widespread, your blood pressure also rises between beats, when your heart is resting, to cause more damage. This sets up a vicious cycle and increases the workload of the heart.

## Artery-health checklist

- **Check food labels,** and select foods with the lowest content of trans-fats (sometimes labelled as partially hydrogenated polyunsaturated fats).
- **Don't re-use oils** or overheat them so that they smoke while cooking, as this promotes oxidation.
- **Add garlic towards the end of cooking** to retain most benefit.
- **If you smoke, quit.**
- **Try to lose excess weight.**
- **Take regular brisk exercise** – at least 30 minutes per day (and preferably 60).

## Foods that can help

- **Eat plenty of fruit, vegetables, beans and nuts** for the antioxidants they contain.
- **Increase intake of folic acid** and vitamins $B_6$ and $B_{12}$, which lower levels of homocysteine – a harmful amino acid that damages artery lining

# What causes it? ATHEROSCLEROSIS IS LINKED WITH:

- increasing age • family history • smoking • being overweight • diabetes
- high blood pressure • poor diet

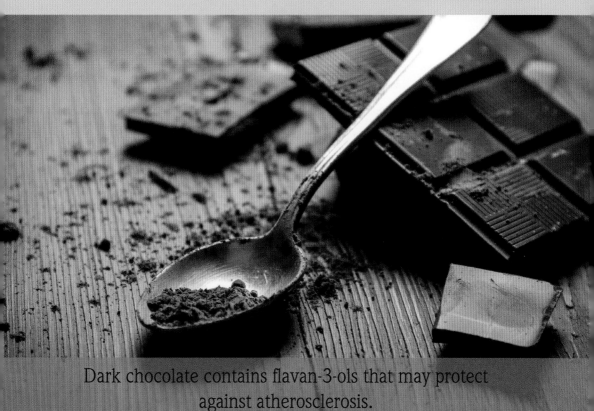

Dark chocolate contains flavan-3-ols that may protect against atherosclerosis.

to hasten atherosclerosis. Foods rich in these include fortified cereals, dark green leaves (such as kale, spinach), wholegrains, oily fish, meats, nuts, avocado, eggs and yeast extract.

- **Treat yourself to dark chocolate:** this contains flavan-3-ols that have been shown to improve platelet function and have been suggested to protect against atherosclerosis.

- **Eat more tomatoes:** tomatoes contain antioxidant lycopene and substances in the 'jelly' around the seeds that reduce platelet stickiness. The higher your tomato intake, the lower the risk of arterial thickening. Cooked tomatoes release more of these beneficial components than eating them raw, so use them in soups, stews and sauces.

## USEFUL SUPPLEMENTS

- **Garlic tablets** have been shown to increase the elasticity of the aorta and to reduce (even partially reverse) atherosclerosis, as well as reducing calcification of arterial walls
- **Tomato extracts** contain antioxidant lycopene and a substance that reduces platelet stickiness
- **Vitamin D** and **magnesium** are needed to process calcium, thus rendering it less likely to contribute to hardening of the arteries (especially important if you take calcium supplements)
- **Folic acid** and **vitamins B$_{12}$ and B$_6$** lower homocysteine levels and may protect against atherosclerosis
- **Turmeric** contains antioxidants that reduce the formation of cholesterol plaque on artery walls
- **Ginkgo biloba** improves peripheral circulation and can help where atherosclerosis causes poor blood flow to the legs and calf pain on exercise

- **Spice up your cooking:** garlic and ginger reduce platelet aggregation and have a relaxant effect on artery walls to improve blood flow. Spices such as turmeric and chilli contain antioxidants with beneficial dilating effects on the circulation.

# Foods to avoid

- **Eat less salt** to improve your blood pressure.
- **Cut back on fat intake** – and choose healthier oils (*see* Fat Facts below).

### FAT FACTS

Most dietary fats contain a blend of saturates, monounsaturates and polyunsaturates in varying proportions. In general, saturated fats tend to be solid at room temperature, while monounsaturated and polyunsaturated fats tend to be oils.

Eating too much saturated fat has been blamed for raising blood

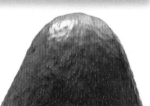

| SELECT OILS RICH IN MONOUNSATURATES | SELECT OILS RICH IN OMEGA-3s | CUT BACK ON OILS RICH IN OMEGA-6s |
|---|---|---|
| macadamia, hazelnut, almond, olive, avocado, rapeseed | fish, macadamia, avocado, walnut, flaxseed | safflower, grapeseed, sunflower, corn, cottonseed, soybean |

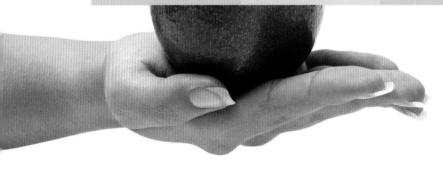

cholesterol levels and triggering atherosclerosis. However, evidence increasingly suggests that it is eating too many omega-6 polyunsaturated fatty acids and not enough omega-3 polyunsaturated fatty acids or monounsaturates which increases your risk of atherosclerosis. Trans-fats are especially harmful. These are formed when polyunsaturated oils are partially hydrogenated to solidify them in the manufacture of cooking fats and margarines. These increase 'bad' LDL-cholesterol, lower 'good' HDL-cholesterol and increase inflammation. As a result, margarines and low-fat spreads are now being reformulated to reduce their trans-fat content. So, when using fats, try to select healthy options rich in monounsaturates and omega-3s (*see* table opposite).

 **Chickpea Masala**

1 tbsp olive or rapeseed oil
1 red onion, chopped
thumb-sized piece of fresh ginger, grated
1 tsp turmeric
1 tsp garam masala
1 tsp ground cumin
2 mild red chillies, sliced
4 cloves garlic, chopped
4 large tomatoes, chopped
(or 1 x 400 g/14 oz can)

1 tbsp tomato purée
zest and juice of 1 lemon
400 g (14 oz) can cooked chickpeas, rinsed and drained
300 ml (½ pt) water
200 g (7 oz) baby spinach leaves, washed
freshly ground black pepper

**(serves 4)**

• Sauté the onions in a wok until soft. Stir in the ginger, turmeric, garam masala, cumin and chillies, and cook over a low heat for a few seconds.
• Add all the remaining ingredients except the spinach, and simmer gently for 10–15 minutes.
• Finally, add the spinach and tamp down into the masala, so it wilts. Season with black pepper to taste.

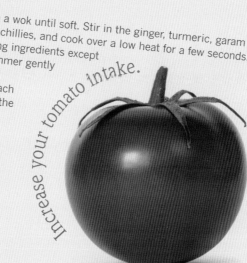

*Increase your tomato intake.*

# Stress

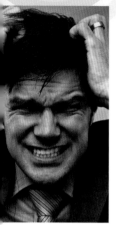

**Stress is a modern term for** when you are under more pressure (either real or perceived) than you are able to cope with at a particular time. These days, increasing numbers of us suffer from it, but eating low-GI foods can help.

Everyone has a different stress threshold, and this depends on what else is going on in your life. When you're fit, well fed and rested, and happy in your relationships, for instance, you can cope with more pressure than when you are unfit, have missed a meal or have stayed up all night arguing.

The symptoms of acute stress result from adrenaline hormone, which mobilizes energy and prepares your body to fight or flee – the 'fight or flight' response. During the second stage, energy would ordinarily be consumed by vigorous exercise through the action of fighting or fleeing, which neutralizes the stress response. Nowadays, however, the need to fight or flee rarely occurs, so the effects of stress can build up, draining your energy and making you feel physically and mentally exhausted. This can ultimately lead to burnout or a nervous breakdown. Stress can also worsen pre-existing health conditions (such

| LOW-GI FOODS eat freely | MEDIUM-GI FOODS eat in moderation | HIGH-GI FOODS go easy |
|---|---|---|
| Bran cereal | Brown rice | Parsnips |
| Baked beans | Wholewheat pasta (cooked al dente) | Baked potatoes |
| Most fruit and vegetables, including sweet potato, carrots, mangoes, kiwi fruit, peas, grapes, oranges, apples, pears, berries | Honey | Cornflakes |
| | New potatoes (boiled) | Raisins |
| | Dried apricots, dates, figs | Doughnuts |
| | Banana | Bread |
| | Potato crisps/chips | Potatoes (mashed) |
| | Sweetcorn | |
| | Porridge oats | |
| | Muesli | |

## What causes it? STRESS IS LINKED WITH:

- change • inability to control situations • pressing deadlines • personality type
- excessive stimulation (noise, light, temperature extremes, overcrowding)

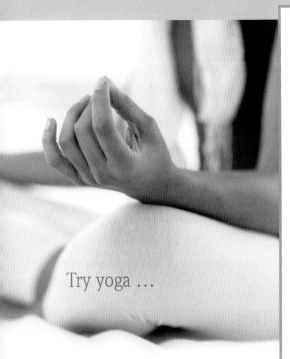

Try yoga ...

## Stress-busting checklist

- **Keep a stress diary** so you can identify and analyse stressors.
- **Think positively** – if you think you can deal with a stressful situation, you're more likely to succeed.
- **View challenges as an opportunity** rather than a threat – and if you do fail, welcome the chance to learn from your mistakes. It's all about taking control.
- **Accept valid criticism** without taking it personally – use it as an opportunity to improve.
- **Accept compliments** without downplaying your achievements.
- **Take regular exercise** – a brisk walk neutralizes the effects of stress hormones. You will feel refreshed, less tense, and work more efficiently as a result.
- **Try yoga** to calm your body and relieve anxiety.
- **Consider counselling,** psychotherapy or cognitive behaviour therapy if difficulties persist.

as eczema, psoriasis and irritable bowel syndrome) and contribute to lowered immunity, low sex drive, indigestion, high blood pressure, heart attack and stroke.

## Foods that can help

Stress raises blood glucose and fat levels, ready to fuel muscles during fighting or fleeing. So, when you're stressed, it's best to select foods with a low to moderate glycemic index (GI), to help maintain an even blood glucose level (*see* table opposite).

Go for lean meats, fish, wholegrains, fruit and vegetables, and eat a nutritious breakfast including bran-based cereals, porridge or muesli with fruit, unsweetened yogurt/fromage frais and skimmed or semi-skimmed milk.

## Foods to avoid

Go easy on foods with a high GI and, if you do eat them, combine small amounts with foods that have a lower

GI, to help even out fluctuations in blood glucose levels (*see* table on page 36). Other things you should monitor include:

## CAFFEINE

The immediate effect of this stimulant drug is to reduce tiredness through a direct action on the brain, which increases alertness and decreases perception of effort and fatigue. However, caffeine also acts on the adrenal glands to increase circulating levels of the stress hormones adrenaline and cortisol. Excess caffeine makes you irritable and jittery, as well as interfering with sleep.

Aim to have no more than one cup of caffeinated coffee per day, and no more than three mugs of not-too-strong tea (preferably green or white tea). If you can, slowly switch to decaffeinated brands, or drink herbal teas such as antioxidant-rich Rooibos, calming camomile or soothing mint. (If you

currently drink lots of caffeine-containing drinks, cut back gradually, over the course of a week, to avoid withdrawal symptoms such as restlessness, irritability, insomnia and headache.)

## ALCOHOL

Avoid excess alcohol – stick to recommended safe intakes. Ideally, alcohol intake should not exceed 2–3 units a day for women and 3–4

## DID YOU KNOW?

**Units of alcohol vary** from country to country, so be sure to refer to the national recommended guidelines where you live. In the UK, for example, one unit is 8 g of pure alcohol, while in the US a standard drink is 14 g alcohol, and in Australia and New Zealand it's 10 g.

Aim to have no more than one cup of caffeinated coffee per day.

## Tzatziki with Crudités

250 ml (8½ fl oz) low-fat Greek-style
natural bio yogurt
half a cucumber, chopped
handful of fresh mint leaves, chopped
1 clove garlic, crushed
zest and juice of 1 unwaxed lemon
freshly ground black pepper

**For the crudités:**
Selection of raw vegetables cut into
finger-sized pieces (such as
carrot, celery, pepper, courgette,
mangetout, broccoli, cauliflower)

(serves 4)

- Place all tzatziki ingredients in a food processor and blitz until smooth.
Season with black pepper to taste. Chill in the fridge for at least one
hour, then serve with the crudités as a dip.

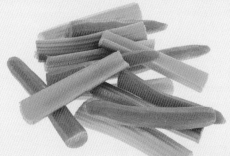

units a day for men, according to UK
guidelines. Aim to have at least two
alcohol-free days per week, too, so that
you're drinking no more than 14 units
per week if you're female, and no more
than 21 units per week if you're male.

The amount of alcohol contained
in beer and wine varies, so check the
strength of what you're consuming, if
possible, and bear in mind that bars
and pubs often serve large measures.
(For example, a small 100 ml/3½ fl oz
glass of wine that is 10 per cent alcohol
in strength contains one UK unit.)

## USEFUL SUPPLEMENTS

- **B group vitamins** – these are depleted during
  times of stress, and deficiency can contribute
  to fatigue
- **Valerian** helps to relieve anxiety, muscle tension
  and promotes tranquillity and restful sleep
- **Rhodiola** reduces anxiety and stress, and has
  an energizing action to overcome stress-related
  fatigue and exhaustion
- **Korean ginseng** is stimulating and restorative,
  improving physical and mental energy, stamina,
  strength and alertness
- **Siberian ginseng** has similar actions to Korean
  ginseng but is less stimulating

# Obesity & weight problems

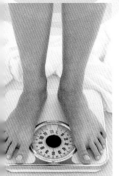

**One in three people in the** Western world is classed as overweight, and an estimated one in four as obese. Carrying excess weight is associated with significant health risks (obese people die, on average, seven years earlier than those of a healthy weight), so keeping your weight down is vital.

You are classed as overweight if you are more than 10 per cent over your ideal weight for your height, and obese if you are more than 20 per cent over. Heredity is a significant factor: if both your parents are obese, you have a 70 per cent chance of obesity too, compared with less than 20 per cent if both parents are lean, as your genes, family eating habits and activity patterns are good predictors of weight gain.

Being overweight or obese results from a long-term imbalance between the amount (and types) of energy sources you eat, and the amount you burn to fuel your metabolism and physical activity. Body-fat stores can be estimated with

## Diet checklist

- **Don't give up** – all diets will work if you stick with them.
- **Drink a glass of water before eating** to avoid mistaking thirst for hunger.
- **Chew each mouthful for longer,** so your brain has more time to receive signals that you're becoming full.
- **Pause regularly when eating,** so your meal lasts longer, and stop when you feel sufficiently full.
- **Keep a food diary** and write down everything you eat – especially helpful when you have difficulty losing weight.

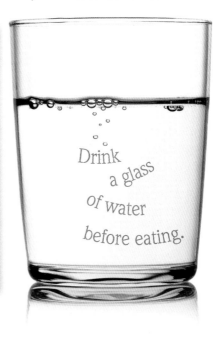

Drink a glass of water before eating.

# What causes it? BEING OVERWEIGHT IS LINKED WITH:

• heredity • age • inactivity • over-eating • alcohol intake • some hormone imbalances

$$BMI = \frac{WEIGHT\ (kg)}{HEIGHT\ (m) \times HEIGHT\ (m)}$$

This gives you a number, which is interpreted as follows:

| BMI | WEIGHT BAND |
|---|---|
| under 18.5 | underweight |
| 18.5 to 24.9 | healthy weight |
| 25 to 29.9 | overweight |
| 30 to 39.9 | obese |
| 40 or greater | morbidly obese |

Alternatively, for a quick guide, just read off your weight and height on the chart below, to discover your BMI weight band

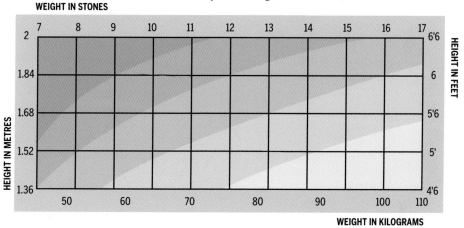

the Body Mass Index (BMI), a widely used tool to gauge if a person is within their healthy weight range (*see* table above). BMI is calculated by dividing your weight (in kilograms) by your height in metres squared.

BMI calculations, however, can be misleading in certain circumstances (body builders with an unusually high muscle mass can have a BMI of up to 30 without being obese, for example).

Researchers have now found that your waist size is a better indicator of health than either your weight or your BMI, as fat stored around your middle increases your risk of developing type 2 diabetes, heart attack or a stroke. You have a higher risk of health problems if:

• you are male and your waist size is more than 94 cm (37 in)
• you are female and your waist size is more than 80 cm (31½ in)

## DID YOU KNOW?

**Losing 10 kg** (22 lb) in weight can lower blood pressure by 10/20 mmHg, reduce fasting blood glucose levels by 50 per cent, blood levels of triglyceride fat by 30 per cent, total cholesterol levels by 10 per cent and 'bad' LDL-cholesterol by 15 per cent (while increasing 'good' HDL-cholesterol by at least 8 per cent).

Regardless of your overall weight, try to avoid becoming too big around the middle, especially as you get older.

## Foods that can help

Insulin is the main fat-storing hormone in the body, and is released when your blood glucose levels rise. Select foods with a low glycemic load that impacts on blood sugar levels as little as possible. Eat fruit, vegetables, salads and wholegrains rather than processed white carbohydrates. Lean meats and beans provide protein that quickly triggers satiety (*see also* table on page 36).

### DIET OPTIONS

Whatever eating pattern you choose, it's important to stick with it until you reach a healthy weight for your height. Always take a multivitamin and mineral supplement to guard against nutritional deficiencies when cutting back on food intake.

- **Low-fat diets** restrict your total fat intake to less than 30 per cent of energy intake, with a focus on reducing saturated (animal) fat, typically to less than 7 per cent daily energy. Moderate consumption of monounsaturated fats (olive and rapeseed oils) is encouraged, as are wholegrain carbohydrates, but refined and simple sugars are avoided. After six months, average weight loss is around 5 kg (11 lb) but after eighteen months, followers typically gain 0.1 kg (¼ lb) from their starting weight.
- **Low-calorie diets** provide 1,000 to 1,500 kcals per day. After six months, average weight loss is around 6.5 kg (14 lb). However, some weight is usually regained and, after eighteen months, followers tend to maintain an overall average weight loss of just 2.3 kg (5 lb).
- **Very-low-calorie diets** typically provide between 400 and 800 kcals per day, in the form of fortified, sweet or savoury drinks that replace between one and three meals a day. Under professional supervision, these diets can help you lose 13–23 kg (29–51 lb) over twelve to eighteen weeks. In the long-term, they are more successful than a traditional calorie-controlled or low-fat diet for keeping weight off. The latest version involves restricting your calories to 500–600 per day for just two days per week, and eating as much as you like (healthy, sensible choices!) for the remaining five days of the week.
- **Low-carbohydrate, high-protein diets** severely restrict carbohydrate initially, then slowly

reintroduce it. Weight loss is rapid and, when the diet is followed for at least four weeks, is typically 2 kg (4½ lb) greater than with diets supplying a higher percentage of energy from carbohydrate. In studies lasting more than twelve weeks, weight loss was 6.56 kg (14½ lb) greater. The long-term benefits are still uncertain and they remain controversial.

- **Low-glycemic diets** provide around 40 per cent carbohydrate (in a wholegrain form that has minimal impact on blood glucose levels) and also limit fat to around 30 per cent energy intake. In a study in which people ate a target of 1,966 kcals per day, those following a low-glycemic diet lost, on average, around 10 kg (22 lb) weight compared with around 6 kg (13¼ lb) in those following a high-glycemic diet. Despite aiming to eat the same, those on the low-GI diet felt fuller and ended up eating a lot less than those on the high-GI diet.

## Foods to avoid

- **Avoid stodgy, sugary, fatty foods** such as doughnuts, cakes, biscuits, pastries and sweets.

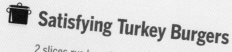

### Satisfying Turkey Burgers

2 slices rye bread
400 g (14 oz) turkey breast, minced
4 shallots, sliced
handful fresh herbs (such as parsley, thyme, coriander), chopped

1 clove garlic, crushed
1 large egg, beaten
freshly ground black pepper

(serves 4)

- Moisten the rye bread with water, and squeeze out any excess. Combine all ingredients, season with black pepper and blitz in a food processor.
- Form into four burgers and grill, or barbecue, until cooked through. Serve with a large mixed salad.

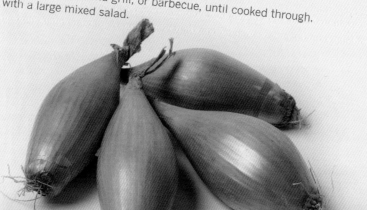

# High cholesterol

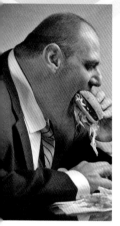

**Although cholesterol has a bad name**, you need a certain amount for healthy cell membranes and to make bile acids, vitamin D and steroid hormones such as oestrogen and testosterone. The key is to reduce the 'bad' kind and increase the 'good' kind ...

Cholesterol is a waxy substance made in your liver (a small amount is also obtained 'pre-formed' from animal-based foods). There are two main types of cholesterol particle in your circulation, which differ in the relative size and weight of the lipoproteins they contain. Low-density lipoprotein (LDL) cholesterol forms tiny, light particles that are associated with hardening and furring-up of the arteries (*see* atherosclerosis, page 32). LDL-cholesterol is therefore known as 'bad' cholesterol.

In contrast, high-density lipoprotein (HDL) cholesterol forms large, heavy particles that are too big to seep into artery walls. HDL is referred to as 'good' cholesterol, as it stays in your circulation and transports 'bad' LDL-cholesterol away from your arteries and back to the liver for processing.

The optimal level for cholesterol is not clear cut, but as a general guide you want:
- a total cholesterol of less than 5 mmol/l (millimoles per litre of blood)
- a 'bad' LDL-cholesterol of less than 3 mmol/l
- a 'good' HDL-cholesterol greater than 1 mmol/l for men or 1.2 mmol/l for women – the higher the better

If your risk of a heart attack is high, the recommended total cholesterol level is below 4 mmol/l, with an LDL-cholesterol of less than 2 mmol/l.

## DID YOU KNOW?

**For every 1 per cent** reduction in your LDL-cholesterol level, your risk of a heart attack reduces by 2 per cent. And, for every 1 per cent rise in your HDL level, your risk of a heart attack also falls by as much as 2 per cent.

## Cholesterol checklist
- **Exercise regularly** – this raises HDL- and lowers LDL-cholesterol.
- **Try to lose any excess weight.**
- **Steam, boil, grill, bake or poach food** rather than frying.

## What causes it? HIGH CHOLESTEROL IS LINKED WITH:

- family history ● poor diet ● lack of exercise ● central (abdominal) obesity
- underactive thyroid gland

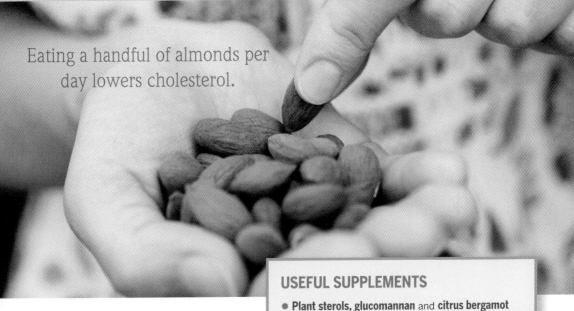

Eating a handful of almonds per day lowers cholesterol.

## Foods that can help

- **Eat plenty of fruit, vegetables and beans.** These provide fibre (which reduces cholesterol absorption), plant sterols (which block cholesterol absorption) and antioxidants (which protect circulating fats from oxidation). It is mainly oxidized cholesterol that is associated with furring-up of the arteries.
- **Eat more wholegrains, nuts and seeds,** which have a beneficial effect on cholesterol balance. Eating 3 g or more of soluble oat fibre per day (roughly equal to two large bowls of porridge), for example, can

## USEFUL SUPPLEMENTS

- **Plant sterols, glucomannan** and **citrus bergamot extracts** can significantly lower cholesterol by blocking its absorption, and can be used with statin medication
- **Garlic extracts** can reduce LDL-cholesterol levels by an average of 11 per cent
- **Lecithin** helps increase the ratio of beneficial HDL-cholesterol to LDL-cholesterol
- **Oat bran** and **psyllium husk** bind cholesterol and other fats in the bowel to reduce LDL-cholesterol
- **Fenugreek** helps to lower total and LDL-cholesterol without affecting HDL levels
- **Red yeast rice** lowers cholesterol in the same way as statin drugs by reducing its production in the liver
- **Co-enzyme Q10** may help to reduce statin-associated muscle side effects of weakness or aches (statin drugs switch off production of both cholesterol and Co-Q10 in the liver)

## GET IT CHECKED

One in ten people with a raised cholesterol level has an undiagnosed underactive thyroid gland. Their slowed metabolism means cholesterol breakdown declines, although their cholesterol production continues as normal. If diagnosed, treatment with thyroxine hormone can reduce cholesterol levels by as much as 40 per cent.

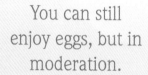

You can still enjoy eggs, but in moderation.

## DID YOU KNOW?

**Research involving over** 100,000 men and women shows that eating an egg a day does not increase the risk of heart disease – even if your cholesterol level is raised.

significantly lower total blood cholesterol levels.

- **Eat foods fortified with sterols/ stanol** (such as margarine and yogurts), as these help to block cholesterol absorption.
- **Cook with garlic:** eating more garlic may not win you many friends, but provides allicin, which helps to lower cholesterol.
- **Go nuts:** eating a handful of almonds per day, or an avocado, significantly lowers total cholesterol levels, due to the monounsaturated fats they provide. In addition, select oils rich in monounsaturated fats (olive, rapeseed or nut oils).
- **Use skimmed or semi-skimmed milk,** rather than whole milk products.
- **Reduce red meat:** aim to eat it no more than once or twice a week, and select lean cuts and trim off visible fat. Instead, have more fish and vegetarian meals that include pulses and beans for protein (as well as fibre and antioxidants).

You can still eat foods such as eggs that contain pre-formed cholesterol, as long as you eat them in moderation. In most people, they raise LDL-cholesterol levels only minimally, as they also provide antioxidants, lecithin and minerals that have a natural cholesterol-lowering action.

# Foods to avoid

Cut back on sources of pre-formed cholesterol (*see* right). The usual advice is to limit your intake of cholesterol to no more than 300 mg per day, which is about the amount found in one egg yolk. If your cholesterol is very high, you may be advised to limit intakes to 200 mg per day. Your liver makes around 800 mg cholesterol per day from some types of saturated fat, so go easy on butter and meat fats.

(NOTE: If you're on statin medication, check the product information leaflet; grapefruit juice interacts with some statin drugs to increase their blood levels, so may need to be avoided.)

| FOOD | CHOLESTEROL per 100 g |
|------|----------------------:|
| Pig liver | 700 mg |
| Lamb kidney | 610 mg |
| Caviar | 588 mg |
| Lamb liver | 400 mg |
| Chicken liver | 350 mg |
| Calf liver | 330 mg |
| Prawns | 280 mg |
| Pheasant meat | 220 mg |
| Butter | 213 mg |
| Squid | 200 mg |
| Duck meat | 115 mg |
| Lobster | 110 mg |
| Hard cheese | 100 mg |
| Chicken dark meat | 105 mg |
| Red meat | 100 mg |
| Chicken light meat | 70 mg |

## 🍲 Healthier Chicken Nuggets

oil spray (olive or rapeseed)
1 large free-range egg, whisked
2 tbsp Dijon mustard
2 handfuls rolled oats
1 handful chopped almonds

1 tbsp Herbes de Provence
freshly ground black pepper
400 g (14 oz) chicken breast, skinned and cut into bite-sized pieces

- Preheat the oven to 200°C/400°F/Gas 6. Spray a non-stick roasting tray with oil.
- Whisk together the egg and mustard in a small bowl. Blitz the oats in a food processor until coarsely ground, then pour into a large sealable food bag with the almonds and herbs. Season well with black pepper.
- Dip each chicken piece in the egg/mustard mix, one at a time, then drop into the bag of oat mix and shake. When all the nuggets are in the bag, seal and shake well to ensure all pieces are coated.
- Remove the nuggets and arrange on the roasting tray. Bake for 20–30 minutes, or until juices run clear. Serve with a large mixed salad and a dressing made from almond, walnut or avocado oil, lemon juice and garlic.

# Diabetes

**Diabetes occurs when blood glucose** levels rise above the normal range. One in ten adults worldwide lives with diabetes and numbers are increasing, although many people remain undiagnosed. Diet helps to prevent type 2 diabetes – even eating an apple a day is protective.

Type 1 diabetes tends to affect people under the age of forty, while type 2 commonly affects those over forty who are overweight, but can occur earlier, even in obese children. Normally, glucose levels are tightly controlled within narrow limits. If too low, your liver makes extra glucose; if too high, your pancreas releases insulin hormone. Insulin acts as a key, moving glucose from the circulation into muscle and fat cells where it is burned as fuel or stored as glycogen (a starch) or fat.

## Caution

If you are taking diabetes medication, don't let glucose levels go below 4 mmol/l, or you may develop a 'hypo', with light-headedness, sweating, trembling, weakness and confusion.

| SYMPTOMS | TYPE 1 DIABETES | TYPE 2 DIABETES |
|---|---|---|
| Excessive thirst | yes | not usually |
| Excessive drinking | yes | not usually |
| Weight loss, despite hunger and increased eating | yes | no – weight gain and obesity are more common |
| Tiredness, listlessness and fatigue | yes | possible |
| Feeling unwell | often | not usually, but can occur |
| Recurrent infections such as cystitis, thrush and boils | often | often |
| Blurred vision | often | not usually, but can occur |

## What causes it? DIABETES IS LINKED WITH:

**Type 1:** family history ● early weaning onto cows' milk ● viral infections
**Type 2:** family history ● obesity ● inactivity ● poor diet ● certain prescribed drugs (such as corticosteroids) ● smoking

One in twenty people with diabetes has type 1, which is associated with a loss of insulin-making cells in the pancreas. Why this occurs is not fully understood. Most people with diabetes have type 2, in which some insulin is made, but not enough to meet your needs. Often insulin levels are higher than normal, at least initially, as cells no longer respond to its effects. This problem, known as insulin resistance, is largely associated with lack of exercise, excess weight and obesity.

The body normally maintains a tight control on your blood glucose level, keeping it within the narrow limit of around 3.9–5.6 mmol/l. Before type 2 diabetes develops, there is a phase in which blood glucose levels are higher than normal (prediabetes with a fasting blood glucose of 5.6–6.9 mmol/l). Once fasting blood glucose rises to 7 mmol/l or more, diabetes is diagnosed.

## Diabetes checklist

- **Try to lose excess weight:** if you have type 2 diabetes and are overweight, losing 10 kg (22 lb) excess fat can reduce your fasting blood glucose levels by 50 per cent.
- **Take more exercise:** exercise improves insulin sensitivity through an effect on fat cells, and increases the amount of glucose burned in muscles.
- **If you smoke, quit!** Smoking is a recognized risk factor for developing type 2 diabetes, and greatly increases your risk of complications such as high blood pressure, atherosclerosis, heart disease and stroke.
- **Monitor your glucose levels regularly.** Your doctor will tell you the target blood glucose levels to aim for, especially if making significant changes to your diet and lifestyle.
- **Wear medical alert ID,** if taking medication, to assist paramedics should you become ill.

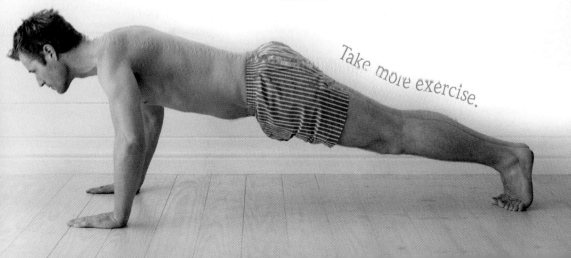

*Take more exercise.*

Persistently raised glucose levels attack blood-vessel linings, causing damage throughout the body. Complications such as loss of vision, kidney failure, heart attack, gangrene or stroke occur more quickly if you also have a poorly controlled high blood pressure, raised cholesterol or triglyceride levels, or if you smoke cigarettes (*see also* diabetes checklist on page 48).

## USEFUL SUPPLEMENTS

- **Multivitamin and mineral supplements** reduce the risk of diabetes-associated infections
- **Chromium, magnesium** and **selenium** may improve glucose tolerance and insulin resistance if you are deficient
- **Cinnamon** and **Korean ginseng** may improve glucose tolerance through an effect on insulin receptors
- **Conjugated linoleic acid** can improve insulin resistance in fat cells
- **Co-enzyme Q10** may improve the function of insulin-producing cells within the pancreas
- **Vitamin C** reduces damage caused by raised glucose levels (**note:** *vitamin C affects HbA1c blood tests and urinary glucose tests, so tell your doctor if taking it*)
- **Alpha-lipoic acid** increases the uptake of glucose into muscle cells and helps to protect against nerve and kidney damage
- **Bilberry extracts** protect the eyes against complications including diabetic retinopathy and cataracts
- **Pine bark extracts** (Pycnogenol) and Ginkgo biloba improve circulation through tiny blood vessels, and may improve insulin resistance

# Foods that can help

- **Replace some carbohydrates in your diet** with healthy monounsaturated fats (such as in olive oil, avocado, almonds, macadamia nuts) and omega-3 fatty acids (from oily fish and walnuts, for example).
- **Follow a wholegrain, high-fibre, low-GI, Mediterranean-style diet** with plenty of fruit, vegetables, berries, fish and olive oil. Even though fruit contains natural sugars, most have a low to moderate glycemic index and do not raise blood glucose levels excessively (though don't over-indulge in dried fruits).
- **Eat an apple a day:** in a study involving 38,000 women, those eating at least one apple a day were found to be 28 per cent less likely to develop type 2 diabetes than those eating none.

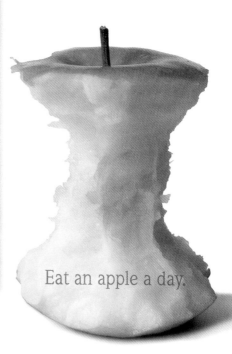

Eat an apple a day.

- **Eat more plums and grapes.**
  Preliminary research suggests plums can improve insulin sensitivity of fat cells and decrease blood glucose levels. Red and black grapes contain protective antioxidants that appear to boost pancreatic insulin production in type 2 diabetes, and protect against kidney damage.

In addition, dark chocolate, cocoa powder, cinnamon, ginger, fenugreek, turmeric, cumin, coriander, mustard seed and curry leaves all have some evidence for improving glucose control.

## Foods to avoid

- **Cut back on foods that contain rapidly digested carbohydrates** and which cause large swings in blood glucose levels, such as sugar, biscuits, cakes, doughnuts, cornflakes, pastries, white bread and potatoes.
- **Go easy on foods with a high GI** – and, if you do eat them, combine small amounts with foods that have a lower GI to help even out fluctuations in blood glucose levels (*see* page 36). Glycemic index values for almost 2,000 foods can be found at www.glycemicindex.com, from the University of Sydney.

## DID YOU KNOW?

**Males who are obese** are seven times more likely to develop type 2 diabetes than those of a healthy weight. For obese women, the risk is twenty-seven times greater.

### Stewed Fruits

3 red-skinned eating apples, cored and chopped
6 ripe plums, halved, stoned and chopped
handful of seedless red/black grapes, halved
1 tsp ground cinnamon
1 star anise
zest and juice of 1 lemon
stevia (optional)

**(serves 4)**

- Place the fruit, spices and lemon juice/zest in a pan and simmer gently, stirring, until tender (5–8 minutes). Discard the star anise.
- Sweeten to taste (if required) with stevia – a natural sweetener with zero calories and no effect on blood glucose levels.

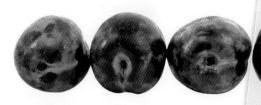
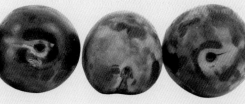

# High blood pressure

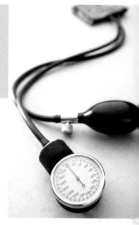

**You need a certain pressure in your** circulation to keep blood moving around your body, but when this pressure becomes too high it increases the risk of serious illness, including heart or kidney failure and stroke. Adjusting your diet can significantly reduce your blood pressure.

Your blood pressure (BP) readings consist of two numbers. The higher number is the systolic pressure in your arteries when your heart contracts. The lower number is the diastolic pressure in your arteries when your heart rests between beats. As BP is measured according to the height of a column of mercury it could support, the units are written as millimetres of mercury (mmHg). An ideal blood pressure reading is between 90/60 mmHg and 120/80 mmHg.

| BLOOD PRESSURE CATEGORY | BP (mmHg) |
|---|---|
| OPTIMAL | Between 90/60 and 120/80 |
| PRE-HYPERTENSION | Between 120/80 and 139/89 |
| HYPERTENSION | 140/90 or above, consistently |

If your top number is 140 or more, or your bottom number is 90 or more, you may have high blood pressure regardless of the other number.

## Why is hypertension harmful?

Your BP varies naturally throughout the day and night in response to emotions and physical activity. When you have hypertension (high blood pressure), however, your BP remains high all the time, even at rest. One in every three adults has high blood pressure, and it becomes more common with age, so that two in every three people over the age of sixty-five are affected.

Hypertension is often called the silent killer, as it causes few symptoms, even if dangerously high. High pressure damages artery linings to hasten hardening and furring-up of the arteries (atherosclerosis). Your heart has to work harder to pump blood through increasingly stiff, non-elastic arteries, so your risk of heart-pump failure and heart attack increases. Damaged blood vessels also increase your risk of a stroke, loss of vision, kidney failure,

## What causes it? HYPERTENSION IS LINKED WITH:

- increasing age • family history • smoking • drinking too much alcohol • stress
- lack of exercise • being overweight • unhealthy diet

dementia, poor circulation (peripheral vascular disease) and, for males, erectile dysfunction.

Although this all sounds rather frightening, the good news is that early diagnosis and treatment can control your blood pressure before it harms your health.

## Foods that can help

The Dietary Approaches to Stop Hypertension (DASH) trials showed that you can significantly reduce your blood pressure within eight weeks by eating:

**More:** fruit, vegetables, wholegrains, poultry, fish, and low-fat dairy products
**Less:** red meat, fats, cholesterol-rich foods and sugary sweets

This approach increases your intake of potassium, a mineral that helps to flush excess sodium from the body through the kidneys. Potassium-rich foods include bananas, avocado, sweet potatoes (with skin), Brussels sprouts, spinach, broccoli, plain low-fat yogurt, beetroot and beet leaves, celery, beans and lentils, parsley and sage.

### DID YOU KNOW?

**It takes at least** one month for salt receptors on your tongue to adjust and detect lower salt concentrations. If food tastes bland, add black pepper, herbs and spices for flavour instead. Lime juice helps your taste buds detect salt.

- **Increase omega-3s:** salmon, mackerel, tuna, sardines, flaxseed, pumpkin seeds and sunflower seeds not only boost your intake of the omega-3 essential fatty acids, but are also good sources of potassium.
- **Drink beetroot juice** – a glass a day can significantly lower blood pressure in some cases, as it contains high levels of nitrites, which help to dilate blood vessels.
- **Try hibiscus tea:** research from the American Heart Association suggests that drinking this three times a day can significantly lower blood pressure.
- **Try pomegranate juice:** researchers from Queen Margaret University,

If food tastes bland without salt, add black pepper, herbs and spices for flavour instead.

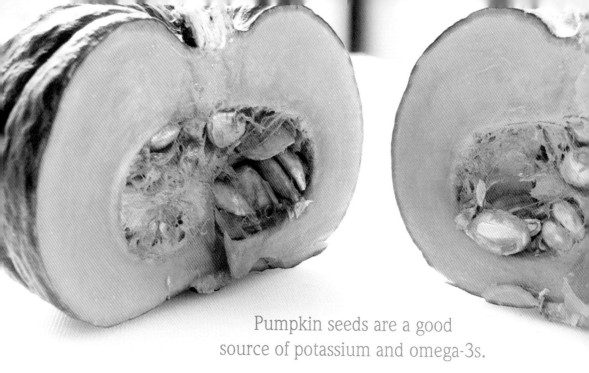

Pumpkin seeds are a good source of potassium and omega-3s.

Edinburgh, have shown that drinking pomegranate juice every day for four weeks significantly reduces blood pressure.

## High BP checklist

- **Lose excess weight** – even losing a little can make a difference.
- **Keep active** – exercise on most days.
- **Stop smoking:** combined with high blood pressure, smoking dramatically increases your risk of heart or lung disease.
- **Reduce stress** – meditation or relaxation therapies can help.
- **Have your BP checked annually.**
- **Take vitamin D** – inadequate levels are a risk factor for high blood pressure.

## Foods to avoid

- **Reduce salt intake:** table salt (sodium chloride) promotes fluid retention in the circulation to increase blood pressure. Reducing salt intake involves more than just not reaching for the salt shaker – you also need to check food labels for sodium. In general, per 100 g (3½ oz) of food (or per serving, if a serving is less than 100 g):

**0.5 g** sodium or more is **a lot** of sodium
**0.1 g** sodium or less is **a little** sodium

Also eliminate high-salt foods such as salted crisps, processed meats (for instance, ham, bacon, salami and hot dogs), cheese, spreads, packet sauces, gravies and ready meals.

- **Reduce processed grains and eliminate sugars** – avoid refined and starchy carbohydrates like white bread, pasta, rice, potatoes and flour products such as pastries, cakes, biscuits and crackers.
- **Avoid sweets, fizzy drinks and chocolates,** as these raise levels of insulin, which is now known to act on the kidneys to increase blood pressure.
- **Avoid caffeinated drinks** as far as possible, as these can also have a negative impact on blood pressure.
- **Drink sensibly:** although one or two units of alcohol are relaxing and

## DID YOU KNOW?

**Mindfulness meditation** and transcendental meditation can significantly reduce hypertension.

beneficial, too much increases blood pressure. Limit your daily intake (no more than two or three units for women, and three or four for men) and have regular alcohol free days, too. Track the number of units you drink at www.drinkaware.co.uk.

 **Beetroot, Walnut & Herb Dip with Pitta Crisps**

250 g (9 oz) pack cooked beetroot
1 small bunch each of coriander & parsley
50 g (2 oz) shelled walnuts
1–2 cloves garlic, crushed
3 tsp extra virgin olive oil
2 tsp red wine vinegar
freshly ground black pepper

For the pitta crisps:
1 pack brown pitta bread
olive oil for brushing
freshly ground black pepper

(serves 4)

- Preheat the oven to 180°C/350°F/Gas 4.
- Roughly chop the beetroot and herbs and put in a food processor with the walnuts and garlic, and process to a coarse paste.
- Add the oil and vinegar and season generously with freshly ground black pepper. Taste to check the seasoning – you may need to add a little more vinegar if the beetroot are particularly sweet. Set aside for the flavours to mingle while you make the pitta crisps.
- For the pitta crisps, slice each pitta into 2–3 strips diagonally and gently prise each strip in half. Arrange on baking sheets, brush with the oil and season with freshly ground black pepper. Bake in the oven for 10–15 minutes or until the pitta strips are dry and crispy. The crisps will keep in an airtight tin for at least a week.

*From www.lovebeetroot.co.uk*

# Coronary heart disease

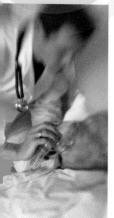

**One in three heart attacks** is linked with an unhealthy diet. If the coronary arteries supplying blood to your heart become narrowed, heart muscle cells may not receive all the oxygen they need, leading to coronary heart disease (also known as coronary artery disease).

Your heart contracts and relaxes around seventy times a minute – that's 100,800 times per day and over 2.76 billion times during an average lifespan. As it is continually active, it needs more fuel and oxygen than any other muscle in your body. Poor blood supply causes heart muscle to cramp when starved of oxygen. This leads to angina, which feels like a tight pressure, heaviness or dull ache behind the breastbone, which may spread into the neck, jaw or down the left arm. Angina typically comes on during exercise and fades within a few minutes of resting.

When the blood supply to your heart is compromised more severely (for example by a blood clot), prolonged lack of oxygen causes heart muscle cells to die, which is known as a heart attack. Heart attack pain is similar to angina, but can come on at any time and is unrelieved by rest. It also usually lasts longer, is more intense and may be accompanied by sweating, paleness, dizziness or shortness of breath. The 'Hollywood heart attack', in which the victim grimaces and clutches their chest, is less common in real life. Often, a heart attack is heralded by feelings of fatigue, indigestion or chest discomfort (rather than pain) and an urgent need to empty the bowels. In older people, a heart attack may cause few symptoms except extreme tiredness or a 'funny' feeling.

## Heart-health checklist

- **Exercise regularly** for at least 30–60 minutes on most days, to keep your heart fit.
- **Lose any excess weight,** especially the 'menopot' around your waist (carrying extra weight increases the workload of your heart).
- **Stop smoking:** tobacco damages artery linings and hastens a heart attack.
- **Avoid excess stress.**
- **Keep alcohol intake within recommended limits,** as too much causes dangerous heart rhythms.
- **Know your blood pressure and cholesterol levels,** and maintain tight control of existing risk factors such as high blood pressure, diabetes and raised cholesterol (through diet, lifestyle and any necessary prescribed medication).

## What causes it? CORONARY HEART DISEASE IS LINKED WITH:

• family history (mother having a heart attack before age sixty or father before age forty-five) • smoking • sedentary lifestyle • poorly controlled high blood pressure or diabetes • high cholesterol • obesity • stress

### Don't delay!

The weak link in surviving a heart attack is delay in seeking treatment. If you think you could be having a heart attack, call an ambulance immediately. Chew an aspirin (to help dissolve any blood clots), lie down and try to stay calm.

Eating oily fish can help protect against harmful heart rhythms.

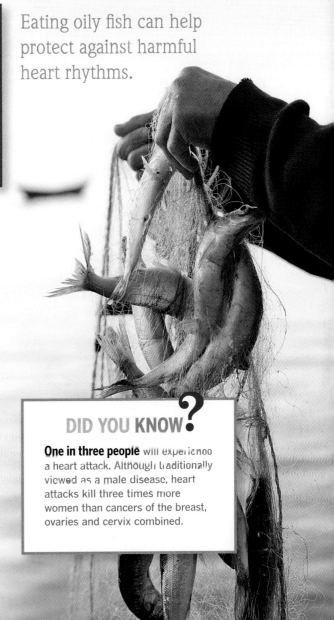

### Foods that can help

• **Eat more wholegrains, fruit, vegetables, beans, nuts and seeds** – one in three heart attacks is linked with an unhealthy diet containing too many processed foods and excess refined carbohydrates (especially sugar and white flour).
• **Select monounsaturated and omega-3 fats** found in olive, rapeseed, avocado, walnut, almond and macadamia oils.
• **Eat more oily fish** (such as salmon, sardines, mackerel, herring; *see also* page 28). These contain omega-3, which helps to lower triglycerides (a harmful type of circulating fat), prevents unwanted blood clots and protects against harmful heart rhythms.
• **Choose healthy snacks** such as fresh or dried fruit and unsalted

### DID YOU KNOW?

**One in three people** will experience a heart attack. Although traditionally viewed as a male disease, heart attacks kill three times more women than cancers of the breast, ovaries and cervix combined.

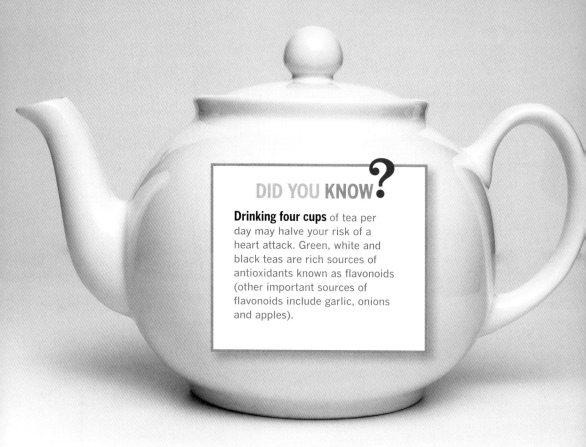

## DID YOU KNOW?

**Drinking four cups** of tea per day may halve your risk of a heart attack. Green, white and black teas are rich sources of antioxidants known as flavonoids (other important sources of flavonoids include garlic, onions and apples).

nuts instead of crisps or sweets. Eating oats, nuts and beans helps to lower cholesterol levels.
- **Opt for wholegrain bread, rice and pasta** rather than refined 'white' versions.

### MEDITERRANEAN MAGIC
A study published in the *New England Journal of Medicine* found that following a Mediterranean diet supplemented with extra virgin olive oil (participants were given 1 litre/ around 2 pints per week!) or tree nuts (30 g/1 oz of walnuts, almonds and hazelnuts daily) reduced the risk of a

heart attack or stroke by almost one third, compared with a traditional low-fat diet (none were asked to cut calories). Participants were also allowed up to seven glasses of wine a week, but discouraged from soft drinks and pastries.

Aim for the magic 'five a day' (or preferably more) of fruit, vegetables and salad items, for the beneficial fibre, vitamins, minerals, antioxidants and plant hormones they provide. People who regularly eat tomatoes and tomato products, for example, are less likely to develop heart disease than those who eat them infrequently.

## Foods to avoid

- **Cut back on cakes,** biscuits, pastries, fried foods, butter, cream, lard and full-fat milk or cheese, to maintain a healthy weight.
- **Keep processed meats to a minimum,** and eat red meat (trimmed of excess fat) no more than once or twice a week.
- **Remove skin** from chicken and turkey.
- **Avoid salty foods** and don't add salt during cooking or at the table (*see* high blood pressure, page 52).

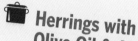

## Herrings with Olive Oil & Almonds

4 tbsp olive oil
4 herring fillets, deboned
4 sprigs fresh rosemary, chopped
1 bay leaf
1 lemon, sliced
bag of mixed salad leaves or rocket
handful of flaked almonds

**(serves 4)**

- Sauté the herring, rosemary, bay leaf and sliced lemon in olive oil for 8 minutes, or until the fish is cooked through. Drain the fillets. Serve on a bed of salad leaves, sprinkled with flaked almonds.

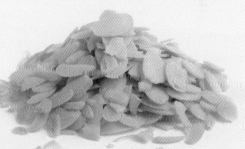

USEFUL SUPPLEMENTS

- **Omega-3 fish oils** reduce blood stickiness, lower blood pressure and protect against abnormal heart rhythms, especially in heart muscle receiving a poor blood supply
- **Krill oil** contains the same beneficial fatty acids as omega-3 fish oil supplement, plus additional antioxidants
- **Vitamin D** may reduce the amount of calcium laid down in artery walls as part of the hardening and furring-up process
- **Magnesium** and **potassium** help to lower blood pressure through direct effects on artery dilation and flushing excess salt from the body
- **Co-enzyme Q10** is vital for energy production in heart muscle cells, helps arteries to dilate, lowers blood pressure, and helps heart muscle pump more efficiently
- **Garlic** helps to lower cholesterol, reduce blood pressure and protects against hardening and furring-up of the arteries
- **Olive leaf extracts** contain thirty times the beneficial polyphenols supplied by extra virgin olive oil to reduce unwanted blood clotting and boost blood flow through coronary arteries
- **Tomato extracts** contain antioxidant lycopene and a substance that reduces platelet stickiness

One in three heart attacks can be linked with an unhealthy diet.

# Stroke

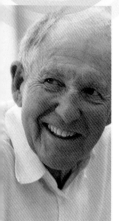

## Act quickly

If you think someone may be having a stroke, call an ambulance. Rapid treatment can help to reduce damage.

**If you live to the age of** eighty-five, you have a one in five chance of experiencing a stroke. The factors that protect against a stroke are similar to those that help to maintain a healthy circulation and protect against a heart attack, as they affect the blood supply to the brain.

A stroke is a sudden loss of control of one or more parts of the body due to a sudden interruption of blood supply to part of the brain. There are three main types of stroke:

- **a thrombosis**, in which a clot forms in a brain artery (this accounts for 45 per cent of cases)
- **an embolism**, in which a clot from elsewhere in the circulation travels in the bloodstream to lodge in the brain (35 per cent of cases)
- **a haemorrhage**, in which a ruptured blood vessel causes bleeding within or over the surface of the brain (20 per cent of cases)

Symptoms and signs vary depending on the part of the brain affected, but usually come on quickly, such as:

- sudden loss of consciousness
- confusion or loss of memory
- loss of movement of one or more parts of the body, usually on one side (for example, left arm, left leg and left side of the face)
- numbness in part of the body
- speech difficulties and difficulty swallowing

For every ten people that die of stroke, four could have been saved if their blood pressure was controlled.

## Stroke-prevention checklist

- **Stop smoking** – smoking doubles your risk.
- **Maintain a healthy weight** to reduce the chance of developing high blood pressure.
- **Exercise daily.**
- **Know your blood pressure, glucose and cholesterol levels** and ensure that they are well controlled.

## Foods that can help

- **Eat a low-GI diet** with more wholegrains and less processed carbohydrates.
- **Get your five-a-day:** obtaining at least five or six servings of fruit and vegetables daily reduces your risk of stroke by up to 30 per cent.
- **Drink pomegranate, grapefruit or orange juice:** a glass a day reduces the risk of stroke by as much as a quarter.

## What causes it? STROKE IS LINKED WITH:

• increasing age • family history • atherosclerosis • high blood pressure • diabetes • raised cholesterol • smoking • excess alcohol • lack of exercise • irregular heartbeat • damaged heart valves • producing too many blood cells (polycythaemia)

**Note:** *a third of strokes are unpredicted, and may result from a congenital weakness or abnormality in the brain circulation, such as a small 'berry' aneurysm.*

• **Eat more fish:** eating fish on a weekly basis reduces your risk of stroke by 12 per cent, with additional reductions of up to 2 per cent per serving per week, as fish oils reduce abnormal blood clotting.
• **Cut back on salt and alcohol intake:** too much of either can lead to high blood pressure.

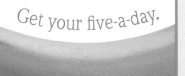

*Get your five-a-day.*

### USEFUL SUPPLEMENTS

• **Vitamin C** – those with high levels are 26 per cent less likely to have a stroke
• **Vitamin D** – those with high levels are half as likely to experience a stroke
• **Selenium** – low selenium levels quadruple your risk of a fatal stroke
• **Calcium, magnesium and Co-enzyme Q10** help to lower blood pressure
• **Garlic** helps lower blood pressure, cholesterol, triglycerides and reduces blood stickiness
• **Folic acid** protects against atherosclerosis
• **Reishi** reduces abnormal blood clotting, and lowers blood pressure and LDL-cholesterol
• **Omega-3 fish oils** reduce blood stickiness and triglycerides

 ## Ruby Red Pomegranate, Apple & Banana Smoothie

100 g (3½ oz) Ruby Red pomegranate seeds
1 medium banana
1 tbsp plain yogurt
200 ml (7 fl oz) freshly pressed cloudy apple juice

• Put the pomegranate seeds in a blender, whizz for 30–40 seconds and strain the juice. Rinse the pomegranate seeds out of the blender and discard.
• Add the banana, yogurt, pomegranate juice and apple juice to the blender and whizz until smooth.

*From: www.rubyredpomegranates.co.uk*

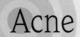

# Acne

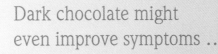

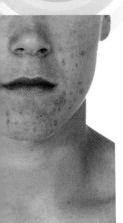

**Although acne is often viewed** as a teenage problem, it is increasingly persisting into adulthood, sometimes only appearing for the first time in later life. Poor diet can worsen symptoms – but chocolate may not be as bad as you think ...

Acne is an inflammatory skin disease due to infection of blocked hair follicles. It occurs when skin glands secrete excessive amounts of oil (sebum) under the influence of androgen hormones. Skin cells also divide more rapidly and may block hair follicles so that sebum is trapped inside. This produces a classic, enlarging blackhead or whitehead. Changes in skin acidity encourage the overgrowth of *Propionibacterium acnes* bacteria, which 'feed' on trapped sebum and trigger inflammation.

There are three types of acne:
- **mild acne**, in which comedones predominate, appearing as whiteheads when closed, or open blackheads
- **moderate acne**, in which inflammatory lesions predominate, with pustules and papules (raised pimples with an underlying deeper infection)
- **severe acne**, in which nodules and cysts develop along with inflammatory papules and pustules, and there is a high risk of scarring

## Acne checklist

- **Take acne seriously** – treatment can prevent permanent scarring.
- **Don't pick spots** – this spreads infection and can produce longer-lasting spots that scar.
- **Look for water-based cosmetics** and skin-care products labelled as 'noncomedogenic'.
- **Ask your doctor** about medication.
- **Persevere** – treatments can take eight weeks or more to work.
- **Request referral** to a dermatologist if your skin doesn't improve.
- **Cosmetic treatments** such as peels, laser therapy and filler injections can reduce scars.

## Foods that can help

Although there's no conclusive evidence that acne is solely caused by a poor diet, it can make symptoms worse. Nutrition influences the effect of male hormones, the 'stickiness' of skin cells and the degree of inflammation that occurs.

Follow a low-GI diet that does not produce swings in blood sugar levels; one study found that males following a low-GI diet for twelve weeks improved twice as much as those following a

## What causes it? ACNE LINKED WITH:

● increased sensitivity of oil glands to androgen hormones ● bacterial secretions leading to inflammation ● overgrowth of skin cell plugs

high-GI diet (twenty-five fewer spots, on average, versus twelve fewer spots). Fruit and vegetables contain anti-inflammatory antioxidants and mostly have a low GI. Oily fish contains omega-3 oils (DHA, EPA) that also reduce inflammation.

### CHOCOLATE

Although it's often claimed that chocolate makes acne worse, there is little evidence to support this. In fact, dark chocolate containing at least 72 per cent cocoa solids might even improve symptoms, as it is one of the richest dietary sources of anti-inflammatory antioxidants.

## Foods to avoid

● **Cut back on sugary and carbohydrate-rich foods:** these promote release of insulin, which enhances the effects of androgen hormones, and increases the proliferation of skin cells.
● **Switch to goat's milk.** Cow's milk contains sugars (such as lactose), growth factors and hormones. Researchers found that, of over 4,200 boys tested, those consuming more than two servings of milk per day were more likely to have acne than those consuming dairy products less than once a week. Try switching to goat's milk and butter instead.

● **Cut back on processed foods:** their vegetable oils (such as sunflower, safflower and corn oils) contain omega-6 fats that promote inflammation in excess.
● **Reduce intake of red meat,** as this contains hormone-like substances that may affect DHT levels in body tissues.

 **Sweet Eve Strawberries with Smoked Salmon & Cracked Pepper**

400 g (14 oz) smoked salmon
200 g (7 oz) Sweet Eve strawberries
1 lemon
freshly ground (or cracked) black pepper

**(serves 4)**

● Spread the smoked salmon in equal portions on four plates. Hull the strawberries and slice them thinly. Cut the lemon lengthways into quarters.
● Scatter the strawberry slices over the smoked salmon, or arrange them in a spiral around each plate. Coarsely grind (or scatter the cracked) black pepper generously over the top. Serve with the lemon wedges.

*From: www.sweetevestrawberry.co.uk*

ACNE **63**

# Eczema

**This common skin problem** affects up to one in five children and an estimated one in ten adults. There are a number of dietary allergens linked with eczema, so paying attention to what you eat is essential.

Eczema is an inflammatory skin disease that typically appears on the hands, inside the elbows or behind the knees, but may be found anywhere on the body. The most common type is atopic, or allergic, eczema, which produces dryness, itching, and scaliness. In severe cases, it may spread to affect most of the body.

Worsening eczema, with blisters and weeping sores that crust, is often associated with a skin bacterium, *Staphylococcus aureus*. If symptoms flare up, seek medical advice.

## Foods that can help

- **Eat a healthy, wholefood diet,** providing at least five – or preferably more – servings of vegetables and fruit per day, for their valuable antioxidant content.
- **Avoid processed foods.**

### DIETARY ALLERGENS

Try eliminating cow's milk (switch to rice milk) or gluten-containing products (found in wheat, barley and rye) for two weeks to see if symptoms improve. If you think you could have gluten sensitivity, see your doctor for a blood test to confirm whether or not you are affected. Ensure a good calcium intake from nuts, seeds, wholegrains, leafy vegetables and supplements, if avoiding dairy products long-term (you may be able to tolerate probiotic yogurt, as the allergens it contains are modified by the beneficial bacteria present). If symptoms don't improve, consult

## Eczema checklist

- **Apply soothing, emollient creams** liberally.
- **Avoid contact with soap,** detergents, cleansers, bubble bath, cosmetics, perfume, solvents, industrial chemicals and household cleaning materials.
- **Wear gloves** for housework, gardening and when preparing citrus fruit, raw vegetables, meat and fish.
- **Reduce stress,** which can cause flare-ups.
- **Contact dermatitis** can be triggered by nickel allergy.

# What causes it? ECZEMA IS LINKED WITH:

● heredity (in atopic eczema, two in three people have a family history of asthma, hay fever or eczema) ● overactive immune responses against certain environmental factors and foods

a nutritional therapist to follow an elimination diet that avoids other common food triggers. Suspect foods are then reintroduced in a particular order to identify which, if any, makes your symptoms worse.

The top twelve dietary allergens linked with eczema are: milk, eggs, wheat, corn, soy, peanuts, tree nuts, chocolate, finfish/shellfish, tomatoes, citrus fruits, berries. Eczema may also occur as an adverse reaction to food additives, especially E104, E214, E215, E216, E218 and E282. Allergenic cross-reactivity can also occur with related plant groups: for example, if you react to apple, you may also react to hazelnut, potato, carrot and celery; and if you are sensitive to latex, you may react to banana, avocado, kiwi, chestnut, soybean, peanut, papaya and fig.

## USEFUL SUPPLEMENTS

- **Probiotic supplements** (non-dairy versions available) may boost immunity and reduce eczema flare-ups, especially in children
- **Evening primrose oil** helps reduce itching and dryness
- **A multivitamin and mineral** may help, as nutrient deficiencies (especially antioxidants and zinc) have been linked with scaly skin rashes
- **Omega-3 fish oils** (assuming you're not sensitive to fish), or **flaxseed** and **algae oils**, can reduce skin inflammation, especially if you also cut back on intake of omega-6 fats found in processed foods
- **Additional antioxidant supplements** (such as vitamins C, E, selenium, pine bark or grapeseed extracts) also help to reduce inflammation

## Quinoa Tabbouleh

400 g (14 oz) cooked quinoa
4 spring onions, chopped
1 clove garlic, crushed
zest and juice of 1 lemon
handful fresh mint leaves, chopped

handful fresh parsley, chopped
freshly ground black pepper
dash of hempseed oil
lettuce and black olives to serve
(optional)

(serves 4)

● Place all ingredients in a bowl and toss together. Chill for 1 hour to allow the flavours to blend. Serve on a bed of lettuce and garnish with black olives, if desired.

# Psoriasis

**Psoriasis is an inflammatory skin disease** that affects around one in fifty adults. Symptoms usually appear between the ages of ten and thirty, although it can occur at any age. Eating oily fish can help.

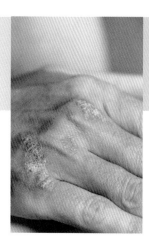

Psoriasis develops when new skin cells are produced around ten times faster than normal. They push up to the surface more quickly than the dead cells they are designed to replace can fall away. As cells accumulate, they form characteristic raised red patches covered with fine, silvery scales. The red, scaly patches (plaques) can vary in size from a few millimetres to extensive areas covering most of the body. In some cases, sterile pustules form – usually on the palms and soles; other sufferers may develop a flaky scalp, and thickening and pitting of the nails. One in five people with psoriasis also develop inflamed joints, known as psoriatic arthritis.

## Psoriasis checklist

- **Try yoga,** meditation or other relaxation techniques, as stress can provoke flare-ups.
- **Don't smoke:** smoking affects immune function and can worsen symptoms.
- **Add Dead Sea mud or mineral salts** to bath water. These contain magnesium, calcium, bromide and zinc that soak into the skin and slow the rate of skin cell production.
- **Try aloe vera gel** (in one study, gel applied three times a day healed over 80 per cent of plaques within four weeks).
- **Apply skin treatments at set times,** so you get into a routine, and leave treated skin uncovered for at least 15 minutes (then put on loose clothing).
- **Apply scalp treatments at least an hour before bed;** wearing a disposable shower cap helps treatment to penetrate.

## Foods that can help

- **Eat more oily fish:** omega-3 fish oils can damp down skin inflammation. Eating oily fish two or three times per week can reduce symptoms: high-dose fish oil supplements (1122 mg EPA and 756 mg DHA per day) were found to reduce psoriasis lesions within four to eight weeks. Itching decreased most rapidly, followed by scaling, and then redness.

Top up your turmeric ...

## What causes it? PSORIASIS IS LINKED WITH:

- heredity • abnormal immune responses • abnormal essential fatty acid metabolism
- food sensitivities

- **Top up your turmeric!** This spice contains curcumin, which can reduce skin inflammation: recent studies suggest it targets cell-signalling pathways involved in skin cell regeneration and wound healing.

## Foods to avoid

- **Cut back on omega-6 fats,** which promote inflammation, found in sunflower, safflower and corn oils, plus many processed foods.

### DID YOU KNOW?

**Exposure to sunlight** can help by synthesizing vitamin D in your skin, which may alleviate symptoms (take vitamin D supplements, especially in winter; selenium supplements may also help).

Some people have found benefit in avoiding foods high in saturated fats, red meats, dairy foods (including cheese), eggs, gluten, alcohol, coffee and refined sugars. (NOTE: If deciding to follow a restricted diet for more than a few weeks, seek nutritional advice.)

 **Baked Salmon with Lemon & Turmeric**

30 ml (1 fl oz) extra virgin olive oil
2 tsp ground turmeric
2 tsp Herbes de Provence
4 x 150 g (5 oz) salmon steaks
freshly ground black pepper
1 unwaxed lemon, thinly sliced

**(serves 4)**

- Preheat the oven to 190°C/375°F/Gas 5. Mix the olive oil with the turmeric and Herbes de Provence.
- Place the salmon steaks on a sheet of foil (large enough to wrap them in). Brush with the herby turmeric mixture and season well with black pepper. Arrange the lemon slices on top.
- Wrap the steaks and bake for 30 minutes, until just cooked through.

# Rosacea

**Temporary facial flushing after a hot drink may be a sign.**

**The usual onset of this** common skin condition is between the ages of thirty and fifty, although symptoms may also occur in the teens. Certain foods and drinks can act as triggers, so adjusting your diet can help to alleviate symptoms.

Rosacea usually starts with temporary facial flushing after eating spicy food, drinking alcohol or hot drinks, or when overly hot. Gradually, the redness becomes more persistent and may become blotchy, or remain diffuse. Visible, thread-like blood vessels (telangiectasia) may also appear. If allowed to progress without treatment, the skin becomes permanently red and acne-like pustules start to appear. Unlike acne, however, blackheads do not form, and the pustules are usually confined to the 'blush' areas of the face, so don't affect the back or chest. Inflammation of the eyelids (blepharitis) and/or conjunctivitis can also occur.

In some people – especially older males – the skin on the nose becomes thickened and red with enlarged follicles. This leads to a bulbous swelling of the nose known as rhinophyma. Rosacea tends to keep coming back over a five- to ten-year period, then often disappears, although any thickened skin changes – such as those on the nose – will remain permanently.

## Rosacea checklist

- **Seek medical advice,** as topical antibiotics can help.
- **Use a non-greasy high-protection sun cream** (SPF 15 or higher), or apply a product that reflects and blocks out ultraviolet rays with titanium dioxide or zinc oxide.
- **Apply aloe vera gel** twice a day – this can reduce inflammation.
- **Use creams containing vitamin K** to treat skin redness and visible small capillaries, or try pulsed intermittent light or laser therapy.

## Foods that can help

Some people find it helpful to follow an alkaline diet that avoids acid-forming foods. Although some fruits, such as oranges, lemons, limes and tomatoes, are acidic to taste, the way they are processed in your body actually uses up acid. Fruit, vegetables and salads are therefore the main alkaline-forming foods in the diet. For sweetness, use stevia

## What causes it? ROSACEA IS LINKED WITH:

- heredity • sensitivity of tiny blood vessels in facial skin • abnormal immune reactions
- possibly an infection of oil glands with bacteria or a skin mite (*Demodex folliculorum*)

## DID YOU KNOW?

**Rosacea affects around** 1 per cent of the population, but some estimates suggest as many as one in ten middle-aged women are affected.

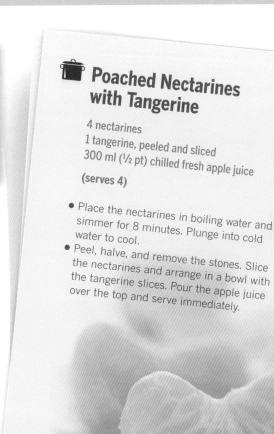

### 🍲 Poached Nectarines with Tangerine

4 nectarines
1 tangerine, peeled and sliced
300 ml (½ pt) chilled fresh apple juice

(serves 4)

- Place the nectarines in boiling water and simmer for 8 minutes. Plunge into cold water to cool.
- Peel, halve, and remove the stones. Slice the nectarines and arrange in a bowl with the tangerine slices. Pour the apple juice over the top and serve immediately.

(a natural sweetener), honey, maple syrup or agave syrup instead of sugar. And make sure you drink plenty of water.

Following an alkaline diet means cutting out some grains (barley, oats, quinoa, rice, wheat), dairy products (cheese, milk, ice cream, yogurt), animal proteins (eggs, poultry, meats, seafood), beer and wine. These foods are important sources of protein, vitamins and minerals, however, so it's best to follow a strict alkaline diet under the supervision of a medical nutritionist, to guard against any dietary deficiencies.

## Foods to avoid

As a general guide, try to avoid spicy foods, coffee, tea, sodas, and foods with preservatives, colourings, artificial sweeteners and other additives.

# Asthma

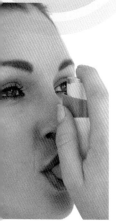

**This inflammatory disease of the** lungs affects an estimated one in ten children and one in twelve adults in the Western world. But did you know that coffee can reduce airway spasms, or that balancing your intake of dietary fats could help?

People with asthma have airways that are red, swollen and inflamed, making them overly sensitive to a variety of triggers. During an attack, the airways go into spasm, producing symptoms of coughing, wheezing, tightness and shortness of breath. As the attack progresses, the lining of the airways swells and produces excess mucus, which often causes a second bout of tightness and wheezing six to eight hours later.

## Foods that can help

- **Consume more omega-3s.** Asthma has been linked with an imbalance in dietary fats, so aim to increase your intake of omega-3s, found in oily fish such as mackerel, herring and salmon (*see also* page 28), wild game meat such as venison

Grass-fed beef contains omega-3s.

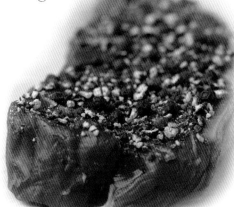

---

## Asthma checklist

- **Always take medications as prescribed** – asthma can be life-threatening.
- **Seek medical advice** if you wake with symptoms, your peak-flow readings are poor, you have to use your reliever inhaler more than once a day, or if you have to make compromises in your life because of symptoms.
- **Avoid smoky places** and don't let anyone smoke in your home or car.
- **Keep your home dust-free** – dust with a damp cloth and use a vacuum with a special filter.
- **Use anti-dust-mite covers** on your bedding.
- **Learn the Buteyko method of breathing** from an accredited trainer.
- **Maintain a healthy weight:** obesity increases inflammation in the body, including the lungs.

## What causes it? ASTHMA IS TRIGGERED BY:

**Allergic asthma:** pollens • house dust mites • animal fur • fungal spores • certain foods such as peanuts, eggs and milk products **Non-allergic asthma:** viral infections • cigarette smoke • cold or damp air • exercise • strong emotions • stress • cosmetics • perfume • air pollution • volatile chemicals • hormonal changes • some drugs

and buffalo, grass-fed beef, omega-3 enriched eggs and omega-3 fish oil supplements. At the same time …

- **Reduce intake of omega-6 vegetable oils** (safflower, grapeseed, sunflower, corn, cottonseed and soybean oils, found in margarines, convenience and fast foods) and replace with healthier oils such as rapeseed, olive, walnut, almond, avocado, hempseed or macadamia oils, which supply good amounts of omega-3s and/or monounsaturated fats.
- **Eat more fruit and veg:** people with a high intake have better lung function and are less likely to develop asthma. Apples and dark green leafy vegetables are especially protective.

- **Increase probiotic bacteria** (found in yogurts and supplements): these may protect against asthma by priming the immune system against allergic responses.
- **Treat yourself to dark chocolate and coffee:** these contain methylxanthines such as caffeine and theobromine, which can suppress cough and reduce airway spasm.

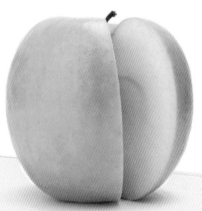

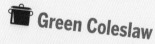 **Green Coleslaw**

1 Granny Smith apple
zest and juice of 2 organic, unwaxed lemons
half a small green cabbage, shredded
2 carrots, grated

**(serves 4)**

1 red onion, thinly sliced
handful fresh herbs, chopped (such as dill or parsley)
150 ml (¼ pt) low-fat natural bio yogurt
freshly ground black pepper

- Grate the apple into a bowl containing the lemon juice and zest. Mix well to stop the apple discolouring.
- Combine with the remaining ingredients. Season well with black pepper, and serve.

# Age-related macular degeneration (AMD)

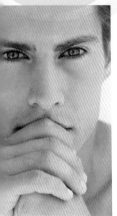

**Most people know that a healthy diet** is good for the heart, but did you also know it's vital for your eyes? Vegetables such as spinach, watercress and sweetcorn provide some protection against this common cause of failing sight as you get older.

Age-related macular degeneration (AMD) is a painless, progressive loss of vision that is most often diagnosed in people over the age of sixty-five, but can start to develop in your forties and fifties. AMD is associated with a loss of yellow pigments in a part of the retina called the macula. These pigments, lutein and zeaxanthin, are sometimes referred to as 'nature's sunglasses', as they protect the macula from the damaging chemical reactions involved in light detection. When levels of these pigments fall, light can damage the macula, leading to a widening circle of visual distortion. Because it affects the centre of your field of vision, it blanks out words so you can't read, and means you can't drive or even recognize someone's face when you look straight at them.

Seek immediate advice if you notice visual distortion of straight lines, as this is often one of the first signs.

## Foods that can help

A good dietary intake of lutein is the mainstay of prevention, as it cannot be made in your body.

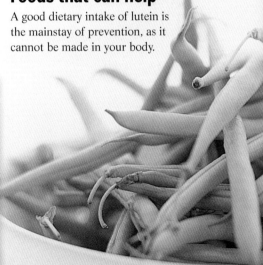

## Eye-health checklist

- **Have regular eye tests** – at least once a year.
- **Wear sunglasses** that carry the UV400 mark to protect your eyes from the sun.
- **If you smoke, quit** – smokers are four times more likely to develop AMD.
- **Eat at least five portions of fruit and veg per day**, including those that are lutein-rich.
- **Consider taking a lutein supplement** as a nutritional safety net as you get older.

## What causes it? AMD IS LINKED WITH:

- increasing age ● family history ● smoking ● poorly controlled high blood pressure
- raised cholesterol ● excessive exposure to strong sunlight ● lack of lutein and
zeaxanthin in the diet

Lutein (and zeaxanthin) is found in orange, yellow, red and dark green fruit and vegetables, plus egg yolk (*see* list below). In addition, tomatoes are protective, as they contain the powerful antioxidant lycopene; high intakes of lycopene can halve your risk of developing AMD (cooked tomatoes offer the greatest benefit). Eating oily fish may also protect against the progression of this age-related condition.

### LUTEIN-RICH FOODS

Aim to eat more of these eye-friendly foods whenever you can:
- kale, spinach, cabbage, chard, watercress
- sweetcorn and green peas
- broccoli and green beans
- yellow and orange peppers
- mangoes, tangerines and oranges
- eggs

 ## Classic Watercress Soup

1 tbsp olive oil
1 small onion, chopped
1 small stick celery, chopped
350 g (12 oz) potato, peeled and diced
600 ml (1 pt) chicken or vegetable stock
3 x 85 g (3 oz) bags watercress
150 ml (¼ pt) milk
pinch of nutmeg
squeeze of lemon juice
salt and freshly ground black pepper

**(serves 4)**

- Heat the oil in a large pan, add the onion and celery and sauté over a medium heat for 5 mins until pale golden. Stir in the potato and stock and bring to the boil. Cover and simmer for 10 minutes, or until the potato is tender.
- Stir in the watercress, cover and cook for a further 5 minutes, or until the watercress is wilted. Transfer the soup to a food processor and blitz until smooth. Return the soup to the rinsed-out pan, add the milk, nutmeg, lemon juice and seasoning to taste. Gently reheat until piping hot and serve with crusty bread.

*From www.watercress.co.uk*

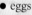

# Cataracts

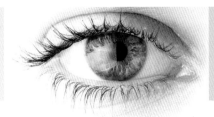

**Carrots may not be able to** make you see in the dark, but they *can* help keep your eyes healthy. Our eye lenses are vulnerable to oxidative damage when dietary antioxidant intake is poor – so eating enough of the right kind of vegetables really can help protect your vision.

## Cataract-prevention checklist

- **Wear sunglasses** to protect your eyes from harmful UV rays. Make sure they offer full UV400 protection. Wrap-around styles help to prevent reflected light from entering at the sides.
- **Make sure children wear sunglasses in bright light,** as their crystal-clear lenses let in more UV light.
- **Wear a wide-brimmed hat** or a baseball-cap when working outdoors, even on cloudy summer days.
- **Consider vitamin C, vitamin E and bilberry extract supplements.** Studies suggest that those taking vitamin C supplements for ten years or more are up to 45 per cent less likely to develop cataracts, while bilberry extracts plus vitamin E were found to stop age-related cataract progression in 97 per cent of cases tested.
- **Have regular eye tests.**

Most people over the age of sixty-five have some degree of cataract, which progresses with age. A cataract is an opacity in the normally crystal-clear eye lens, caused by changes in lens proteins similar to those that turn cooked egg white cloudy. This results in blurring, sensitivity to sun glare, changes in colour perception, and seeing haloes around light.

## Foods that can help

The lenses in your eyes obtain oxygen and nutrients by diffusion from the eye fluids in which they're suspended, so obtaining plenty of antioxidants is vital to help protect against oxidative damage.

## What causes it? CATARACTS ARE LINKED WITH:

● exposure to ultraviolet rays ● smoking ● diabetes ● a career working outdoors ● light-coloured eyes ● laser eye surgery (which thins the cornea) ● taking certain drugs which increase sensitivity to sunlight (such as tetracyclines, phenothiazines, psoralen, allopurinol) ● obesity

People with the highest dietary intakes of antioxidants (vitamins C, E, selenium and carotenoids such as lutein, zeaxanthin and lycopene) are less likely to develop cataracts than those with low intakes. Dark green leafy vegetables (such as spinach, kale and watercress), broccoli, carrots and other yellow-orange fruit and vegetables are especially beneficial, as they contain carotenoid pigments such as lutein and zeaxanthin. Research involving almost 77,500 female nurses found that, after other potential cataract risk factors were controlled for, those with the highest intakes of lutein and zeaxanthin were 22 per cent less likely to develop cataracts severe enough to require removal than those with low intakes.

 ## Roasted Carrot, Spinach & Feta Salad

450 g (1 lb) carrots, peeled and cut into chunks
1 red onion, cut into wedges
1 red pepper, deseeded and cut into wedges
60 ml (2 fl oz) olive oil
3 tbsp pumpkin seeds
1 tsp cumin seeds

2 whole cloves garlic
juice of half a lemon
1 tsp runny honey
freshly ground black pepper
100 g (3½ oz) bag baby spinach leaves
100 g (3½ oz) feta cheese, crumbled
2 tbsp chopped fresh mint leaves

**(serves 4)**

● Preheat the oven to 220°C/425°F/Gas 7.
● Place the carrots, onion, pepper and half the oil in a large roasting tin. Season well. Toss together until everything is coated in oil. Roast for 15 minutes, then stir in the seeds and garlic and roast for a further 10 minutes, until the carrots are just tender but still have a bit of bite.
● Take the vegetables out of the oven and remove the garlic cloves. On a chopping board, slip the garlic from the papery skin and, using the blade of a knife, work it to a smooth paste. Put the garlic paste in a small bowl with the remaining oil, lemon juice and honey, and whisk together with a fork. Season to taste.
● Empty the spinach leaves into a large serving bowl, then add the roasted vegetables, feta, chopped mint and dressing. Toss lightly together until mixed.

*From www.britishcarrots.co.uk*

# Insomnia

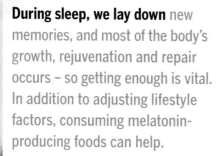

**DID YOU KNOW?**

**You're three times** more likely to develop symptoms when exposed to a common cold virus if you get less than seven hours' sleep a night than if you achieve eight or more.

**During sleep, we lay down** new memories, and most of the body's growth, rejuvenation and repair occurs – so getting enough is vital. In addition to adjusting lifestyle factors, consuming melatonin-producing foods can help.

Insomnia is the subjective feeling of excessive wakefulness, whether from difficulty falling asleep, maintaining sleep or waking unrefreshed. Most people experience insomnia at some stage of their life – usually when they are worried or stressed. Insomnia can last just a few days (for instance, jetlag), from one to three weeks (stress), or last longer term (anxiety, depression, illness or alcohol abuse). People with persistent insomnia are more likely to have a serious accident, and to develop depression, high blood pressure or heart disease.

Adults need, on average, seven to eight hours' sleep per night, but this reduces with age. If you sleep less, but wake feeling refreshed, you are getting all the sleep you need.

## Good-sleep checklist

- **Avoid napping** during the day.
- **Take regular exercise** – but nothing strenuous late in the evening.
- **Avoid substances that interfere with sleep** such as caffeine, nicotine and excess alcohol.
- **Relax before going to bed:** read a book, listen to soothing music or have a bath.
- **Get into a routine** by going to bed at a regular time each night.
- **Make sure your bed is comfortable,** and your bedroom is dark, quiet and warm (a temperature of 18–24°C/65–75°F is ideal).
- **If you can't sleep, get up** – read a book, or write down what is worrying you. When you feel sleepy, go back to bed and try again.

## Foods that can help

- **Eat a healthy, wholefood diet** with plenty of complex carbohydrates (such as cereals, bread, pasta), fruit and vegetables, avoiding overly rich food, especially at night.
- **Eat foods containing tryptophan,** needed for the production of the sleep-inducing hormone melatonin. These include turkey, bananas, oats, honey, wholegrains, dairy products, oily fish, plus some nuts and seeds. A light bedtime snack that includes complex carbohydrates (wholegrains) and low-fat dairy

## What causes it? INSOMNIA IS LINKED WITH:

- stress • anxiety • depression • shift work • bereavement • relationship problems
- unfavourable noise, light or temperature • excess caffeine

products such as semi-skimmed milk or live yogurt, for example, provides calming substances such as magnesium and calcium as well as tryptophan.

- **Drink Montmorency cherry juice:** it's one of the few foods to contain melatonin, and so can help you sleep (also available in supplement form).

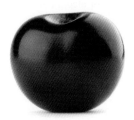

## USEFUL SUPPLEMENTS

- **Valerian** reduces anxiety and helps to improve sleep quality
- **Rhodiola** helps to relieve stress-related fatigue and exhaustion when anxiety is at the root of a sleep problem
- **5-HTP** provides building blocks for making melatonin, and helps you enter the deeper stages of sleep for a more refreshing rest
- **Magnesium** may improve sleep quality where magnesium intakes are low
- **Camomile** has sedative properties and is often included in sleep-promoting herbal teas
- **Lavender** (inhale the essential oil) has relaxing sedative qualities, and is a popular home remedy

## 🍲 Open Turkey Sandwiches

4 slices oated wholegrain bread
a little butter
4 tbsp sour cherry jam or cranberry sauce

250 g (9 oz) cooked turkey breast, sliced
handful fresh spinach leaves

**(serves 4)**

- Spread each slice of bread with a small amount of butter, then a tablespoon of the cherry jam or cranberry sauce. Arrange the turkey and spinach leaves on top, and enjoy.

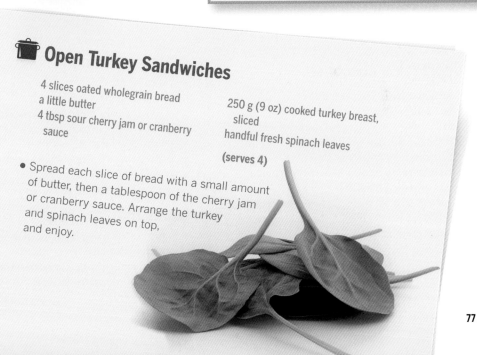

# Depression

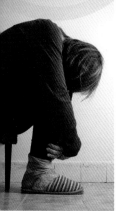

**Few people are blessed with** a happy mood all the time. This is a normal part of everyday life, but if mood dips too low, a full-blown depressive illness can result. Studies show that omega-3s can help improve symptoms – so eating more oily fish could be key.

Depression is a biological illness associated with an imbalance of brain chemicals such as serotonin, noradrenaline and dopamine. These neurotransmitters pass messages from one brain cell to another, and imbalances slow you up both physically and mentally. Typical symptoms include exhaustion, difficulty concentrating, sadness and crying for no apparent reason. Sufferers may comfort eat and gain weight initially, but, as depression

takes hold, they tend to lose their appetite, have difficulty sleeping, and wake early in the morning.

## DID YOU KNOW?

**Your lifetime risk** of a major depressive illness is one in ten if you are male, and one in four if you are female – so get those omega-3s into your diet.

## Depression checklist

- **Seek medical help** if you think you may be depressed.
- **Talk about it:** sharing your thoughts and feelings helps you work things out.
- **Exercise regularly** for at least 30 to 60 minutes, most days, as this releases mood-lifting brain endorphins.
- **Get out into the fresh air** as much as possible.
- **Cultivate your hobbies** and your friends.
- **Avoid excess alcohol** – keep intake within recommended levels.

## Foods that can help

- **Follow a low-GI diet** concentrating on wholegrain cereals, root vegetables, legumes and oily fish. Try not to skip meals, however low you feel.

## What causes it? DEPRESSION IS LINKED WITH:

• heredity • hormone imbalances • childhood trauma • bereavement • lack of vitamin D/sunshine • social isolation • low self-esteem • pessimistic personality • abuse of alcohol, nicotine or illicit drugs • having a serious illness such as cancer, heart disease, diabetes or Alzheimer's

• **Obtain vitamin D** by eating oily fish, liver, fortified margarine, eggs, butter and fortified milk, and from sensible sun exposure, or take supplements.

### OMEGA-3S

Omega-3 fish oils (DHA and EPA) play an important structural and functional role within the brain. Worldwide, populations that eat very little fish have a higher prevalence of depression than in those where fish is eaten regularly. Clinical trials suggest that intakes of 2 g of omega-3 fatty acids can improve symptoms of depression, lengthen periods of remission and improve the short-term course of the illness in those affected.

## Mackerel Kedgeree

400 g (14 oz) cooked brown rice
2 hard-boiled eggs, chopped
3 smoked, peppered mackerel fillets, flaked
4 tbsp fresh parsley, chopped
4 spring onions, chopped
4 tsp garam masala (or freshly ground curry powder)
150 g (5 oz) low-fat fromage frais
small bunch of watercress

**(serves 4)**

• Mix all ingredients except the watercress together. Serve hot or cold, piled onto a platter. Garnish with the watercress.

Get those omega-3s into your diet.

# Seasonal affective disorder (SAD)

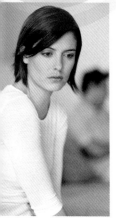

**Also known as SAD,** seasonal affective disorder syndrome affects an estimated 5 per cent of the population. Four times more women are affected than men, and it is most common between the ages of twenty and forty. Getting enough of the right vitamins in your diet is essential.

SAD is a form of depression that comes on when the days shorten and exposure to natural sunlight is reduced. This may be the remnant of a primitive hibernation response. A wide range of symptoms can occur, including tiredness, general slowing down, sleepiness, over-eating and weight loss, plus emotional symptoms such as tearfulness, low self-esteem, depression and social withdrawal. Symptoms tend to last from November to March, with remission during the summer months. A milder form of winter depression – often called sub-syndromal SAD, or winter blues – can also occur, and tends to start around two months later.

SAD usually recurs each year, and the diagnosis is made when someone has had three winters of symptoms (two of which are consecutive), with symptoms improving during the summer months. Some people get a rebound mild hypomania (a form of hyperactivity) in spring and summer, too.

## SAD checklist

- **Try light therapy:** symptoms are often improved by using a special light box that emits bright, cool white fluorescent light (2500 lux), similar to natural daylight. Light therapy is best started a month or so before your symptoms usually develop. Light boxes may work best when timed to come on with increasing brightness before you wake, to simulate a natural dawn.
- **Get up early** rather than lying in bed (which will increase feelings of lethargy).
- **Get out into the open air** for exercise as much as possible.
- **Eat little and often.**
- **Keep warm.**

## Foods that can help

- **Follow a low-GI diet** concentrating on wholegrain cereals (such as porridge, brown rice, pearl barley, quinoa, oatcakes, unsweetened breakfast cereals), root vegetables (carrots, parsnip, turnip, swede, sweet potatoes), cruciferous plants (broccoli, cauliflower, Chinese leaves), legumes (lentils, kidney beans) and fresh or dried fruit.

## What causes it? SAD IS LINKED WITH:

● lack of sunlight ● low vitamin D levels ● seasonal variations in the production of brain chemicals (such as serotonin) and thyroid-stimulating hormone ● increased sensitivity to melatonin (a sedative hormone produced by the pineal gland) ● heredity

● **Eat oily fish and cheese** to obtain tryptophan, a substance needed to make serotonin in the brain.
● **Obtain vitamin D** from foods such as oily fish, fish-liver oils, animal liver, fortified margarine, eggs, butter and fortified milk. Vitamin D is important for mood, and low levels during winter, when daylight hours are reduced, may contribute to SAD.
● **Get plenty of vitamins B$_6$ and C:** foods providing vitamin B$_6$ (wholegrains, soy, walnuts, oily fish, green leafy vegetables, avocado, bananas, walnuts) and vitamin C (for example, citrus, kiwi, berries, sweet peppers) help the production of serotonin.

## Foods to avoid

● **Reduce intakes of alcohol, salt and caffeine.**
● **Don't over-eat:** research suggests people with SAD selectively eat more sweet carbohydrates during the winter months.

 **Sweet Potato Fish Pie**

**For the filling:**
1 bunch spring onions, chopped
500 g (1 lb) mixed fish (such as cod, haddock, salmon, smoked salmon, prawns), cut into chunks
1 tbsp chopped fresh dill or parsley
zest and juice of 1 lemon
1 small carton low-fat crème fraîche
freshly ground black pepper

**For the topping:**
700 g (1½ lb) cooked sweet potato, mashed
50 g (2 oz) mature cheddar cheese, grated

**(serves 4)**

● Preheat oven to 190°C/375°F/Gas 5.
● Mix together all the filling ingredients and season well. Spoon into either a pie dish or four individual dishes. Top with the mashed sweet potato, and sprinkle on the cheddar cheese.
● Bake for 45 minutes, or until the fish is cooked through and the topping is golden.

# Attention deficit hyperactivity disorder (ADHD)

**ADHD is a condition that first appears** before the age of seven. Four times as many boys are affected as girls, and it's estimated to affect up to 10 per cent of children (depending on diagnostic definition used). EFA and common nutrient deficiencies may be a contributing factor.

## ADHD checklist

- **Don't smoke during pregnancy** – this triples the risk of a baby later developing ADHD.
- **Consider evening primrose oil and omega-3 fish oil supplements.**
- **Consider a multivitamin and mineral supplement** to correct common nutrient deficiencies such as vitamins A, B complex, C, D, E and minerals (calcium, magnesium manganese, zinc, chromium, selenium and cobalt).

ADHD is a persistent and severe abnormality affecting psychological development, in which a child is continually inattentive, restless and impulsive, so they are unable to sit down quietly even when overly tired or exhausted. Any stimulation leads to feverish excitement, and attempts to calm the child frequently result in screaming fits and hysteria. Some children improve at puberty, with around 40 per cent 'growing out of it'.

## Foods that can help

- **Follow a nutritious wholefood diet:** studies suggest child behaviour is improved by following a diet containing plenty of fresh fruit and vegetables, and avoiding added sugar, artificial colourings, flavourings, chocolate, monosodium glutamate, preservatives and caffeine. In one study, parents recorded a 58 per cent improvement in behaviour, compared with little improvement in those not on this regime.
- **Increase intake of essential fatty acids (EFAs).** Some children with ADHD are lacking in EFAs, either

ADHD is estimated to affect up to 10 per cent of children.

## What causes it? ADHD IS LINKED WITH:

• family history • male gender • essential fatty acid (EFA) deficiency • exposure to toxins including excess alcohol or cigarette smoke during foetal development

because their diet is deficient, their requirements are higher than normal, or their body cannot process them properly. Encourage consumption of oily fish such as mackerel, salmon, trout and sardines (*see also* page 28), plus nuts, seeds, wholegrains and dark green leafy vegetables.

## Foods to avoid

• **Gradually cut out foods containing white flour, sugar and colourings,** and replace with more nutritious alternatives. Only sweeten food when absolutely necessary, with muscovado sugar (also known as

Barbados sugar), honey or molasses, used sparingly.
• **Try excluding common allergens:** a study found that hyperactive children improved on a diet that excluded allergens such as wheat, corn, yeast, soy, citrus, egg, chocolate, peanuts and artificial colourings and flavours. Hyperactivity ratings dropped by over two thirds, from an average of 25 (high) to an average of 8 (low).

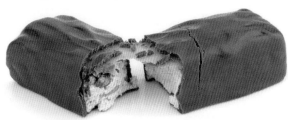

 **Home-made Fishcakes**

400 g (14 oz) cooked, deboned fish (such as cod, haddock, salmon or a mixture), cut into chunks
400 g (14 oz) cooked sweet potato, mashed
zest of 1 lemon, finely grated
1 tbsp fresh parsley, chopped

1 tbsp fresh chives, chopped
freshly ground black pepper
1 omega-3 enriched egg, beaten
handful of fresh brown breadcrumbs
olive, rapeseed or hempseed oil for frying

(serves 4)

• In a bowl, gently combine the fish chunks, mashed sweet potato, lemon zest, parsley and chives. Season with black pepper.
• On a floured board, with floured hands, carefully shape the mixture into four fishcakes. Dip each cake in the egg, making sure all sides are coated, then place into the breadcrumbs, patting the crumbs over until each cake is covered. Chill for at least 30 minutes.
• Fry over medium heat for 5 minutes each side, until crisp and golden.

# Dementia

**More common with increasing age,** dementia affects one in thirty people aged sixty-five to seventy-five, and one in five aged eighty-five and over. But it's estimated that more than half of all cases may be preventable through diet and lifestyle changes.

Dementia is a progressive loss of the ability to think straight. Those affected experience difficulties with language, understanding, familiar tasks, memory and planning, as well as loss of judgement and initiative. Changes in mood, behaviour and personality also occur.

Alzheimer's is the most common type and is linked with an accumulation of altered protein inside brain cells (neurofibrillary tangles) and abnormal protein outside brain cells (amyloid plaques). Dementia with Lewy bodies is associated with the appearance of protein spherules within brain cells, while vascular dementia results from reduced blood flow to the brain. Other, rarer forms of dementia involve a selective loss of brain cells from particular parts of the brain.

While it does become more common with increasing age, it's not considered a disease of ageing, as it is not inevitable.

## Exercise increases blood flow to the brain.

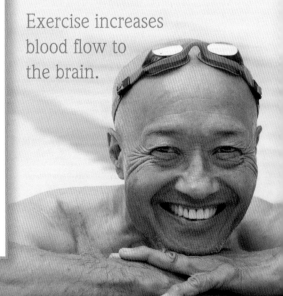

## Dementia checklist

- **Avoid weight gain,** especially during middle age – obesity doubles your risk of dementia.
- **Take regular exercise,** as this increases blood flow to the brain. Those who walk, on average, a mile a day, are half as likely to experience muddled thinking, while those with dementia who walk at least five miles a week experience a slower progression of their condition.
- **If you smoke, quit:** smoking causes spasm of blood vessels and hastens hardening and furring-up of the arteries to reduce brain blood flow.
- **Try therapy:** psychological treatments, behaviour therapy, mental stimulation and reality orientation therapy can help.

## What causes it? DEMENTIA IS LINKED WITH:

• increasing age • family history • smoking • high blood pressure • some infections (such as untreated syphilis) • brain tumours • alcohol abuse • heavy metal poisoning

## Foods that can help

- **Get your five-a-day (or more):** fruit and vegetables contain vitamins, minerals and polyphenols that help to reduce blood pressure and protect against dementia (those with a lower BP are four to five times less likely to develop dementia). Dark green leafy vegetables are especially important as they supply folic acid, which lowers levels of homocysteine – a harmful amino acid associated with arterial damage and dementia risk.
- **Eat fish/seafood at least once a week:** older people with a weekly intake have a lower risk of developing dementia.
- **Obtain vitamin D from your diet.** Vitamin D appears to be directly involved in learning, memory and mood, and may have a protective role in dementia. Sources include oily fish, liver, fortified margarine, eggs, butter and fortified milk.
- **Get a good dietary intake of vitamin E:** this may help to protect against Alzheimer's disease. Dietary sources include wheatgerm oil, avocado pear, butter, margarine, wholegrains, nuts and seeds, oily fish, eggs and broccoli.
- **Step up the soy:** soy isoflavones have an oestrogen-like action and can help improve memory in older women.

 **Avocado & Prawn Cocktail**

4 tbsp low-fat mayonnaise
4 tbsp low-fat crème fraîche
4 tbsp tomato ketchup
squeeze of lemon juice
200 g (7 oz) cooked prawns
handful of fresh baby spinach leaves
2 avocados, sliced
freshly ground black pepper

**(serves 4)**

- Combine the mayonnaise, crème fraîche, ketchup and lemon juice. Add the prawns and mix well.
- Arrange the spinach leaves and avocado slices in four glasses. Top with the prawn cocktail mix, and season with black pepper.

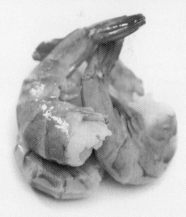

# Endometriosis

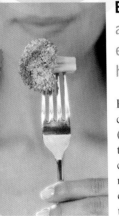

**Endometriosis is one of the most common** gynaecological conditions, affecting as many as one in ten women, although many have mild or even no symptoms. Eating organic food and avoiding red meat can help, while oily fish can alleviate painful symptoms.

Endometriosis is a condition in which cells spread from the womb lining (endometrium) to another part of the body, where they take root and continue to grow. Endometrial cells most commonly transplant to the pelvic or abdominal cavities, but they can also travel further afield, to the lungs, brain and even behind the eyes. Adenomyosis is similar, and occurs when endometrial cells are found within the muscular wall of the womb, nestled between the muscle fibres to form diffuse patches or a lump similar to a fibroid.

Because endometrial cells remain sensitive to the monthly hormone cycle, they may swell and bleed into surrounding tissues once a month to produce pain, inflammation and scarring. Symptoms can include heavy, painful periods, pain during sex and deep pelvic pain (which can occur throughout the menstrual cycle). One in three women also experiences difficulty conceiving.

## Foods that can help

- **Follow a wholefood diet,** avoiding excess salt, caffeine, sugar, fried and processed foods.
- **Go organic:** organic foods contain less of the environmental toxins that mimic the effects of oestrogen hormone.
- **Eat your greens:** research from Italy found that women with the highest intakes of green vegetables and fresh fruit had the lowest risk of endometriosis, whereas those with the highest intakes of beef and other red meat or ham had double the risk of those with the lowest intakes.
- **Eat more oily fish:** women who obtain the most fish oils in their diet have

## Endometriosis checklist

- **Consult your doctor** if you experience heavy, painful periods (one study found an average delay of seven years between onset of symptoms and correct diagnosis).
- **Try pain-relieving medication:** aspirin, paracetamol or ibuprofen can help.
- **Take regular brisk exercise** – this seems to reduce the risk of endometriosis.
- **Drink plenty of fluids** to help maintain optimal hydration and reduce blood stickiness.

## What causes it? ENDOMETRIOSIS IS LINKED WITH:

- heredity • shorter menstrual cycles (less than twenty-seven days) • history of pelvic infection • never having given birth

the least painful menstruation, as essential fatty acids found in fish (and in flaxseed, sunflower, nut and hempseed oils) act as building blocks for hormone-like substances that can improve hormone balance, as well as reducing inflammation and spasm.

- **Increase iodine intake:** lack of iodine has been linked with endometriosis; dietary sources include marine fish and seaweed products.

 ## Salmon Ceviche with Lime & Coriander

225 g (8 oz) ultra-fresh raw salmon fillet, chopped
half a cucumber, peeled and chopped
4 spring onions, chopped
4 handfuls mixed, fresh salad leaves

**For the marinade:**
zest and juice of 4 organic, unwaxed limes
60 ml (2 fl oz) hempseed oil

2 tomatoes, skinned and chopped
1 green chilli, deseeded and finely chopped
handful fresh coriander leaves, finely chopped
2 tsp honey
freshly ground black pepper

**(serves 4)**

- Combine the marinade ingredients. Place the chopped, raw salmon in a non-metallic bowl, pour on the marinade and mix well. Cover and chill for 3 hours, stirring occasionally, until the salmon is opaque.
- Serve as four individual portions, each piled onto a bed of mixed lettuce leaves, and topped with the cucumber and spring onions.

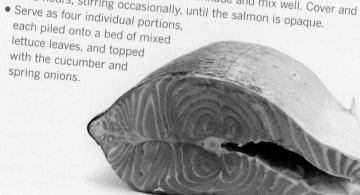

# Painful periods

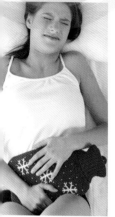

**Painful periods cause discomfort or cramping** just before or during menstruation. One in ten women experience symptoms severe enough to interfere with normal activities. Increasing your dietary intake of omega-3s and magnesium and eating a wholefood diet can help.

Known as dysmenorrhoea, painful periods are more common during the first few years after menstruation has started, and then again as the menopause approaches. They are related to over-production of hormone-like chemicals (prostaglandins) in the lining of the womb (endometrium). These trigger uterine spasms which,

normally, help to close blood vessels and reduce menstrual losses. Excessive painful cramps occur when you make more prostaglandins than usual, or become more sensitive to their effects. The pain of dysmenorrhoea is thought to be linked with lack of oxygen reaching womb tissues during these contractions. As the bowel is also sensitive to prostaglandins, painful periods may be accompanied by diarrhoea, nausea and even vomiting.

Painful periods occurring within two or three years of starting to menstruate have been linked with an unusually narrow cervical canal. This usually improves by the age of twenty-five, and is rare after having a baby.

## Painful periods checklist

- **Try exercising** – this can relieve period pain by encouraging muscles to relax and releasing natural painkillers in the brain.
- **Avoid excess stress,** which makes pain worse.
- **Non-steroidal anti-inflammatory drugs** (such as ibuprofen) reduce prostaglandin production.
- **Consider omega-3 fish oil and pine bark extract supplements** (pine bark can significantly improve menstrual pain when taken for at least two weeks before menstruation).
- **Try magnetic therapy** to relax muscles.
- **Seek medical advice** if symptoms persist, to rule out gynaecological problems.

## Foods that can help

- **Follow a wholefood diet** that avoids excess salt, caffeine, sugar, fried and processed foods.
- **Eat more oily fish:** painful periods are less common in women who eat oily fish regularly, as the omega-3 essential fatty acids they contain have a beneficial effect on the types

## What causes it? PAINFUL PERIODS ARE LINKED WITH:

- young age • narrow cervical canal • a retroverted womb (uterus tilts backwards instead of forwards) • endometriosis • fibroids • pelvic inflammatory disease • polyps • uterine cancer (rarely)

of prostaglandins produced, to reduce muscle spasm.

- **Maximize magnesium intake:** magnesium supplements taken for six cycles were shown to reduce period pains – especially on the second and third days – due to their muscle-relaxant effect. Dietary sources of magnesium include beans (especially soy), nuts, wholegrains (these lose most of their magnesium content when processed), seafood, and dark green leafy vegetables.
- **Cook with ginger** – ginger helps to reduce nausea.

## Foods to avoid

- **Reduce intake of red meat and dairy products.** Some women find this helpful, but – if doing so – ensure you take supplementary iron and calcium to compensate.
- **Cut back on saturated fats.**

 **Ginger-glazed Grilled Salmon**

4 fresh salmon fillets
1 spring onion, chopped

**For the glaze:**
2 tbsp freshly grated ginger
1 tbsp rice vinegar
1 tbsp low-sodium soy sauce
2 tsp honey

(serves 4)

- Combine the ginger, rice vinegar, soy sauce and honey in a bowl. Place the salmon skin-side down in a grill pan, pour on the glaze, cover and leave to soak for 20 minutes.
- Preheat the grill to a medium heat and cook for about 5–10 minutes, until just firm. Garnish with the spring onion.

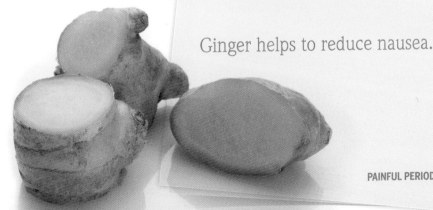

Ginger helps to reduce nausea.

# Premenstrual syndrome (PMS)

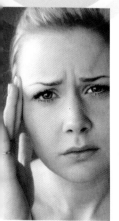

**This common and distressing problem** affects as many as one in two women. But adjusting your diet can bring relief: in one study, dietary changes alone, with no additional medication, gave full relief of severe PMS symptoms in 19 per cent of sufferers.

PMS is a complex of symptoms that begin within the two weeks immediately before a period, and which cease promptly once bleeding occurs. Over 150 symptoms have been described, including anxiety, irritability, increased appetite, sugar cravings, headache, fatigue, low mood, fluid retention, bloating and breast tenderness. The exact cause of PMS is unknown, but it is believed to be linked with a relative imbalance between the two female hormones, oestrogen and progesterone.

## Foods that can help

- **Follow a wholefood diet** with as little pre-packaged convenience foods and additives as possible.
- **Select organic products** when you can, to reduce your exposure to agricultural chemicals that can disrupt hormone balance.
- **Eat a source of complex carbohydrate every three hours** (such as wholemeal bread, rice cakes, digestive biscuits, wholegrain cereals), to keep blood sugar steady; some researchers believe that progesterone hormone cannot bind properly to cell receptors when blood glucose levels are low. In one study, 50 per cent of women gained relief from symptoms, with a further 20 per cent experiencing some improvement.
- **Eat more oily fish,** such as mackerel, salmon, herrings, sardines (*see also* page 28) – their essential fatty

---

## USEFUL SUPPLEMENTS

- **Magnesium** has been shown to improve premenstrual fluid retention (weight gain, oedema, mastalgia, bloating)
- **Calcium and vitamin D** supplements have been shown to reduce headache, negative emotions, fluid retention and pain
- **Evening primrose oil** may help low mood, sugar cravings and breast pain linked with PMS
- **Agnus castus** can relieve a variety of physical and emotional PMS symptoms, including irritability, mood changes, headache and breast fullness

**Note:** *Each supplement tends to help around two out of three women, but must be taken for at least three months to assess the effect.*

acids are needed for optimum hormone balance.

● **Increase dietary intake of calcium and magnesium.** Calcium, found in dairy products, eggs, green leafy vegetables, nuts, seeds and pulses, enhances hormone receptor activity, while magnesium is essential for the activity of over 300 enzymes and is also involved in hormone receptor interactions; dietary sources include nuts, seeds, wholegrains and pulses.

## Foods to avoid

● **Cut down on salt intake** to reduce fluid retention.
● **Cut back on alcohol and caffeine** to reduce irritability and depression.

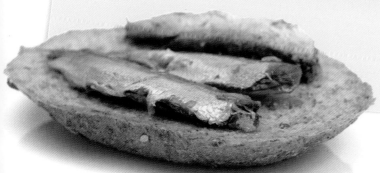

### 🍲 Fresh Sardines on Wholemeal Toast

4 fresh sardines, cleaned
30 ml (1 fl oz) hempseed, rapeseed or olive oil
4 spring onions, sliced
1 clove garlic, crushed
handful fresh herbs, chopped (such as basil or parsley)

8 cherry tomatoes, halved
zest and juice of half a lemon
4 slices wholemeal toast
freshly ground black pepper

**(serves 4)**

● Brush the sardines with the oil and sauté with the spring onion, garlic and herbs until turning golden.
● Add the tomatoes and lemon juice/zest and simmer gently for a further 5 minutes, or until cooked through. Arrange on the toast and season with black pepper.

# Candida

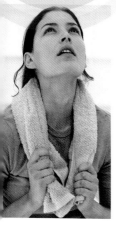

**Candida yeasts are a group of fungi** that live happily in or on the body of just about everyone. Normally, they exist in balance with other micro-organisms, but in the right conditions they proliferate. Many people find that anti-Candida diets improve recurrent symptoms.

Although around eighty different species of Candida exist, only a quarter can cause human diseases. Of these, the most important is *Candida albicans*. Candida thrives best in warm, moist places with an acid pH and a temperature of 20–38°C (68–100°F); these are the usual conditions found in the vagina, some parts of the gut, and in skin creases – especially after vigorous exercise. When conditions are right, Candida yeasts proliferate and put out long, thread-like tubes (hyphae) that burrow between cells. This invasion of local tissues causes redness, soreness, itching and painful swelling. Yeast overgrowth can also produce white clumps which are said to resemble the speckled breast of a thrush – hence the common name.

The presence of Candida in the gut may trigger a hypersensitivity reaction to yeast proteins. This causes the intestinal lining to become 'leaky', so incompletely digested food particles enter the circulation to trigger immune responses. Although controversial, this has been linked with non-specific symptoms such as fatigue, headache, bloating, aches and pains, as well as symptoms compatible with irritable bowel syndrome.

## Foods that can help

- **Follow a low-GI diet** with as few processed foods as possible.
- **Eat plenty of foods that contain natural anti-fungal agents** such as garlic, herbs, spices, nuts (especially coconut) and seeds.
- **Eat an iron-rich diet** (*see* anaemia, page 150) and consume a vitamin C-rich source (such as orange juice) when eating iron-rich foods (such as red meat), as this increases iron absorption from the gut.

## DID YOU KNOW?

**If you need antibiotics**, taking a probiotic supplement helps to maintain intestinal levels of 'friendly' bacteria and may reduce the chance of developing Candida as a side effect.

## What causes it? CANDIDA IS LINKED WITH:

- reduced immunity • antibiotic therapy • raised glucose levels (diabetes) • iron-deficiency anaemia • ultraviolet light exposure • stress

## Candida checklist

- **Wear loose, breathable clothing** and cotton underwear.
- **Avoid getting hot and sweaty** – women may find it helpful to use panty liners that can be changed as necessary throughout the day.
- **Wash underwear at a minimum of 60°C** (hot) or hot-iron to kill Candida spores.
- **Maintain normal, protective levels of acidity** by using specially formulated feminine hygiene products such as pH-balanced gels.
- **Avoid sun beds.**
- **Avoid excess stress** – take time out for rest and relaxation.
- **Try anti-fungal treatments** such as clotrimazole or miconazole cream/pessaries; alternatively, a fluconazole capsule can be taken by mouth.
- **Consider asking your partner to use an anti-fungal cream** if you have recurrent vaginal thrush – men can harbour yeast spores and pass them back without developing symptoms themselves.

Wearing loose clothing can help.

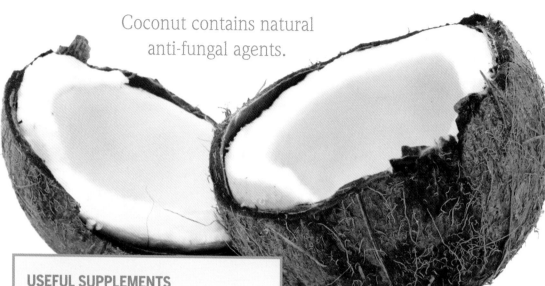

Coconut contains natural anti-fungal agents.

## USEFUL SUPPLEMENTS

- **A multivitamin and mineral** that includes iron will help to guard against nutrient deficiencies
- **Lapacho bark extract** (pau d'arco) is traditionally used to protect against Candida
- **Adaptogens** (such as Siberian ginseng) can be helpful if Candida is associated with excess stress
- **Grapefruit seed extracts, olive leaf extracts** and **caprylic acid** (a fatty acid found in coconut and palm oil, which has a natural anti-fungal action) are all popular anti-Candida remedies

**Note:** *Ensure all supplements, especially B vitamins, are labelled 'yeast-free'.*

- Consume live bio yogurts to replenish intestinal levels of probiotic digestive bacteria that suppress Candida overgrowth in the gut.

## Foods to avoid

Although some people view anti-Candida diets with suspicion, they have undoubtedly helped many people with recurrent, non-specific symptoms. The basic anti-Candida diet is best followed under professional supervision, and involves avoiding products that contain brewer's or baker's yeast, and products that stimulate yeast growth.

- Avoid white or brown sugar and food or drinks containing these (such as honey, jam, desserts, treacle, syrups, cakes, biscuits, sauces, ice cream, soft drinks, dried fruits, milk chocolates, malt, and so on).
- Avoid processed carbohydrates (such as white flour, white rice) and products made from them (biscuits, cakes, buns, white bread). In an ultra-strict anti-Candida diet, intakes of unrefined complex carbohydrates

such as brown rice, wholegrain cereals and wholewheat pasta are also restricted.

- **Avoid products containing yeasts or moulds** such as yeast extracts, cheese, bread made with yeast, alcoholic drinks, vinegar and pickled foods, smoked foods, soy sauce, tofu, grapes and grape juice, unpeeled fruits, dried fruits, frozen or concentrated fruit juices, old and potentially mouldy foods/vegetables, and mushrooms.
- **Avoid some sugar substitutes** such as sorbitol, mannitol, xylitol, aspartame and saccharin, which are metabolized like alcohol to produce substances that can stimulate Candida growth.
- **Avoid alcohol, tea, coffee, cocoa products, malted night-time drinks, fizzy drinks and fruit squashes.** Sometimes dairy products are avoided, too.

If symptoms improve significantly, you are advised to start reintroducing foods one at a time to see which, if any, upset you. If your symptoms are not significantly improved by following a restricted diet, return to eating as wide a range of foods as possible, to guard against any nutrient deficiencies. If you intend to avoid more than a few foods long-term, always seek advice from a nutritional therapist or dietician to prevent nutritional deficiencies.

 **Dairy-free Coconut Yogurt**

250 ml (½ pt) coconut water
450 g (1 lb) coconut, freshly grated
probiotic powder (2 capsules' worth)
vanilla extract or stevia to sweeten (optional)

**(serves 4)**

- Blend the coconut water and coconut flesh until smooth. Add the probiotic powder and briefly blend again. Pour into a jug, cover, and leave at room temperature for the culture to work overnight (around 12–16 hours).
- If you wish, sweeten with vanilla extract or stevia, or add freshly pulped peeled fruit (such as banana) or very dark chocolate, grated. You can also freeze the yogurt to make delicious, probiotic coconut lollies.

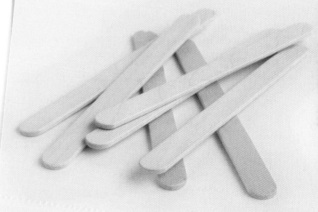

Freeze to make delicious, probiotic coconut lollies.

# Polycystic ovary syndrome (PCOS)

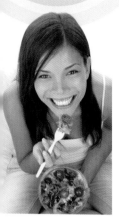

**PCOS affects an estimated** one in four women, although many cases are mild so that, overall, around one in twenty women develop symptoms. Losing excess weight via a low-GI diet can be key to improving symptoms.

As well as producing female hormones, your ovaries normally produce small amounts of male androgens, such as testosterone. If the ovaries produce too many androgens, this blocks the monthly development of egg follicles. The pituitary gland responds by producing more luteinizing hormone (LH) to kick-start the ovaries. As a result, the ovaries enlarge and become covered with multiple small cysts containing under-developed eggs. Symptoms can include periods that become light, irregular or absent, oily skin, acne, excess unwanted hair and difficulty conceiving. Around half of women with symptoms are overweight, with fat mainly deposited around their waist – the male pattern of fat storage also linked with testosterone.

Many women with PCOS also have a metabolic abnormality in which their cells become less responsive to insulin hormone. Women with PCOS are therefore seven times more likely to develop type 2 diabetes than women with healthy ovaries. Researchers are still unsure whether the insulin resistance in PCOS is due to high levels of testosterone, or vice versa, but it looks increasingly like the insulin resistance comes first. Many women with bulimia show evidence of PCOS due to the large fluctuations in blood sugar levels that occur between starving and bingeing.

## PCOS checklist

- **Seek medical advice** if you think you could have PCOS, as treatment is important to maintain a healthy cholesterol, triglyceride and glucose balance.
- **Take regular exercise** to help improve glucose tolerance.
- **If you smoke, quit** – smoking damages the ovaries enough to trigger a menopause at least two years earlier than normal.

## Foods that can help

Even a modest loss of some excess weight (just 6 kg/13 lb) can correct hormone abnormalities, reduce acne and unwanted hair, and improve fertility. In view of the insulin resistance, try to:

## What causes it? PCOS IS LINKED WITH:

● being overweight ● poor glucose handling ● diabetes ● bulimia

● **Follow a low-GI diet** – this involves eating wholegrains, fruit, vegetables, fish and lean meats that have low to moderate effects on blood glucose.
● **Increase intake of isoflavones** (oestrogen-like plant hormones), as these have a balancing effect. These are found in beans, lentils, chickpeas, fennel, nuts and seeds.

### USEFUL SUPPLEMENTS

● **Chromium** is involved in glucose regulation and can improve insulin resistance
● **Agnus castus** or **saw palmetto** extracts can be used to improve hormone balance, but should be taken under the supervision of a medical herbalist

## Foods to avoid

● **Avoid refined carbohydrates** (such as white bread, white pasta and rice, cakes and biscuits), as these promote insulin production.

Eating fennel can help to balance hormones.

## Bean & Fennel Salad

400 g (14 oz) cooked mixed beans
200 g (7 oz) Florence fennel, grated
100 g (3½ oz) carrots, peeled and grated
1 tsp fresh ginger, grated
2 tbsp fresh dill, chopped
2 tbsp fresh parsley, chopped

zest and juice of 1 lemon
2 cloves garlic, crushed
1 tbsp hempseed, rapeseed or olive oil
freshly ground black pepper

**(serves 4)**

● Mix all the ingredients together and marinate in the fridge for several hours before serving.

97

# Infertility

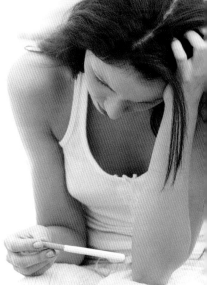

**When trying for a baby**, the average chance of conception is around 20 per cent each month. One in six couples experience difficulty in conceiving, so it's worth giving yourself the best possible chance by eating as healthily as you can.

One in ten couples fail to conceive within the first year.

## Fertility checklist

- **Stop smoking:** men and women who smoke are three times more likely to experience subfertility than non-smokers.
- **Maintain a healthy weight:** women in the healthy weight range are more likely to conceive spontaneously than those who are significantly under or over weight.
- **Avoid stress:** excess stress can disrupt hormone balance, and can even cause loss of menstruation.
- **If you're male, wear loose-fitting cotton boxer shorts;** tight underwear made from man-made fibres can lower sperm count by up to 20 per cent.
- **Take multivitamin supplements designed for pregnancy,** which include folic acid, and avoid any non-essential drugs, herbs and other supplements.
- **Consider using an ovulation predictor kit** to maximize your chances of conception.

Infertility is the inability to conceive. For most people, the term 'subfertility' is more appropriate, as this recognizes that, in most cases, there is still a chance of conceiving naturally, even if the chance is small. A twenty-five-year-old woman will, on average, conceive within five months, while conception tends to take six months or longer for a thirty-five-year old, as fertility reduces with age. Just by chance, one in ten couples fail to conceive during their first year of trying, and 5 per cent fail to conceive within two years.

## Foods that can help

- **Follow a wholefood diet** that is as organic as possible. A low-glycemic diet containing wholegrains rather than refined, processed and sugary foods reduces insulin resistance, which can affect reproductive hormone balance, especially if you are overweight.

## What causes it? INFERTILITY IS LINKED WITH:

- hormone imbalances (including menopause) • low sperm count • producing abnormal sperm or eggs • blocked reproductive tubes • immune reactions • endometriosis • inability to have normal intercourse

- **Select organic fish** – preferably from organic sources to reduce exposure to deep sea toxins such as mercury, PCBs (man-made chemicals) and dioxins.
- **Eat plenty of fresh fruit and vegetables** for vitamins, minerals and trace elements. Pumpkin and other yellow-orange fruit and vegetables provide vitamin A in the form of carotenoid pigments (excess vitamin A in the retinol form – especially from liver products – has been linked with birth defects).

## Foods to avoid

- **Avoid refined, processed and sugary foods.**
- **Avoid alcohol, excess caffeine and fizzy drinks.** Women who drink five or less units of alcohol per week are twice as likely to conceive within six months as those drinking ten units per week or more. 40 per cent of male infertility is linked with just a moderate alcohol intake.

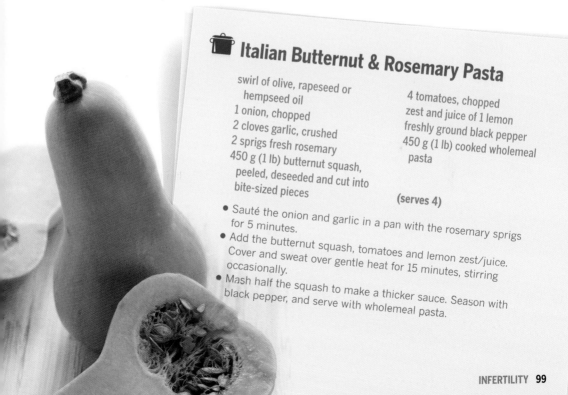

### Italian Butternut & Rosemary Pasta

swirl of olive, rapeseed or hempseed oil
1 onion, chopped
2 cloves garlic, crushed
2 sprigs fresh rosemary
450 g (1 lb) butternut squash, peeled, deseeded and cut into bite-sized pieces

4 tomatoes, chopped
zest and juice of 1 lemon
freshly ground black pepper
450 g (1 lb) cooked wholemeal pasta

(serves 4)

- Sauté the onion and garlic in a pan with the rosemary sprigs for 5 minutes.
- Add the butternut squash, tomatoes and lemon zest/juice. Cover and sweat over gentle heat for 15 minutes, stirring occasionally.
- Mash half the squash to make a thicker sauce. Season with black pepper, and serve with wholemeal pasta.

# Menopause

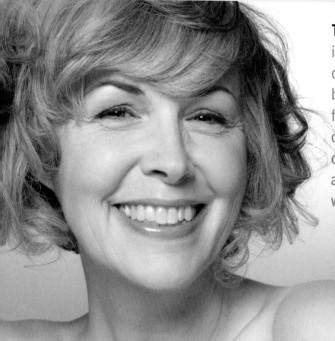

**The menopause is a natural phase** in a woman's life when fertility draws to a close, usually occurring between the ages of forty-five and fifty-five, though it can occur earlier or later. Natural plant hormones can alleviate common symptoms as well as other conditions linked with lack of oestrogen.

The menopause itself is dated from a woman's last period. As the ovaries start to run out of eggs, the levels of female sex hormones – oestrogen and progesterone – fall. Some women notice few problems, but others experience a variety of physical symptoms such as hot flushes, night sweats, intimate dryness, difficulty sleeping, tiredness, headache, pins and needles, joint pains and urinary leakage. Associated emotional symptoms can include mood swings, irritability, difficulty concentrating, anxiety, loss of self-esteem, inability to cope and low sex drive.

In the long term, lack of oestrogen is associated with increased risk of hardening and furring-up of the arteries, high blood pressure, raised cholesterol levels, coronary heart disease and osteoporosis.

## Foods that can help

Many plant foods contain plant hormones (phytoestrogens) that can interact with oestrogen receptors

## What causes it? THE TIMING OF MENOPAUSE IS LINKED WITH:

● age ● heredity ● smoking ● high alcohol intake ● stress ● weight ● medical hormone treatments ● gynaecological surgery

### DID YOU KNOW?

**Pregnancy is still possible** during early menopause, so, if you don't wish to become pregnant, use contraception for at least one year after your last natural period if you're over the age of fifty, or for two years after if you're under fifty. If in doubt, check with your doctor.

to help reduce the risk of various common conditions such as high blood pressure and cholesterol levels, as well as relieving menopausal symptoms like hot flushes and night sweats. The most widely studied are isoflavones, found in soy, chickpeas, lentils and mung beans. Although these are several hundred times less active than human oestrogens, they provide a useful oestrogen boost.

Plant isoflavones are mostly present in an inactive form. Once ingested, bacteria in the large intestine break these down to release the active version. However, isoflavone metabolism varies greatly from person to person, so to ensure you gain the maximum benefit, eat live bio yogurt and take a probiotic supplement with your isoflavones.

To increase your intake of natural plant hormones, aim to eat more:

### Menopause checklist

● **Wear several layers of clothes** that you can peel off during a hot flush.
● **Keep a fan next to your bed** if you need cooling at night.
● **Quit smoking:** smoking reduces oestrogen levels (on average, smokers go through the menopause two years earlier than non-smokers).
● **Avoid excess stress,** which drains the adrenal glands so they are unable to produce their normal tiny amounts of sex hormones to help even out menopausal symptoms.
● **Take regular exercise** for overall fitness.
● **Use a lubricant** to overcome intimate dryness.
● **Consider hormone replacement therapy (HRT)** – this quickly relieves hot flushes and night sweats, but is usually only prescribed for up to five years (counting from the age of fifty) to minimize any associated increased risk of breast cancer.

● **beans** – especially chickpeas, lentils, alfalfa and mung beans, soybeans and soy products
● **vegetables** – dark green leafy vegetables (such as broccoli, spinach, cabbage), exotic members of the cruciferous family (Chinese leaves, kohlrabi), celery, fennel
● **nuts** – almonds, cashew nuts, hazelnuts, peanuts, walnuts and nut oils

- **seeds** – especially flaxseed, pumpkin, sesame, sunflower and sprouted seeds
- **wholegrains** – especially corn, buckwheat, millet, oats, rye and wheat
- **fresh fruit** – including apples, avocados, bananas, mangoes, papayas and rhubarb
- **dried fruit** – especially dates, figs, prunes and raisins
- **herbs** – especially angelica, chervil, chives, garlic, ginger, parsley, rosemary and sage

- **Increase omega-3s:** omega-3 essential fatty acids found in linseeds, hempseeds and oily

fish have been shown to lower cholesterol, improve hormone-related depression, and may help to protect against breast cancer.
- **Drink an extra pint of semi-skimmed or skimmed milk per day** for calcium (ensure vitamin D intake is also good, so that calcium is processed properly).

## Foods to avoid
- **Reduce intake of saturated fat.**
- **Avoid excess sugar and salt;** steer clear of obviously salty foods, and don't add salt during cooking or at the table – use herbs and black pepper for flavour instead.
- **Avoid alcohol, caffeine or spicy foods** if these provoke hot flushes.

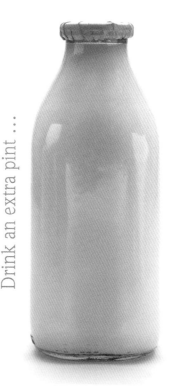

Drink an extra pint ...

---

### USEFUL SUPPLEMENTS

- **Isoflavone extracts** can significantly reduce hot flushes
- **Black cohosh** helps to relieve hot flushes, vaginal dryness, depression and anxiety
- **Sage leaf extracts** can relieve hot flushes and night sweats, and improve memory
- **Evening primrose oil** is a good source of GLA, an essential fatty acid that provides building blocks for making sex hormones
- **Calcium** and **vitamin D** supplements help to improve bone mineral density and can reduce the risk of bone fractures
- **Rhodiola** helps to reduce stress and improves energy levels to help overcome anxiety and fatigue
- **Omega-3 fish oils** can reduce the risk of heart attack
- **5-HTP** provides building blocks for making serotonin in the brain, which, as well as lifting mood, also improves sleep quality

#  Nourishing Vegetable Casserole

2 tbsp olive, rapeseed or hempseed oil
1 large onion, chopped
2 garlic cloves, crushed
1 large leek, washed and chopped
2 stalks celery, chopped
2 carrots, peeled and chopped
4 potatoes, peeled and chopped
1 large parsnip, peeled and chopped
4 large mushrooms, sliced
400 g (14 oz) can cooked chickpeas,
   drained (or a handful of lentils)
1 large red pepper, chopped

1 pack (around 300 g/10 oz ) fresh
   cherry tomatoes, or a 400 g/14 oz
   can chopped tomatoes
2 tbsp flaxseeds
handful fresh herbs (sage, parsley,
   rosemary, oregano), chopped
1 bay leaf
1 tbsp tomato purée
250 ml (½ pt) low-salt stock
freshly ground black pepper

(serves 4)

- Heat the oil in a large pan or casserole dish, and sauté the onion, garlic and leek until soft.
- Add all the remaining ingredients and season with black pepper. If needed, add more water until the vegetables are just covered.
- Bring to the boil, then reduce heat and simmer, stirring occasionally, for 1 hour.

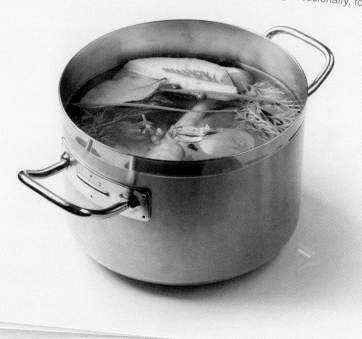

# Osteoporosis

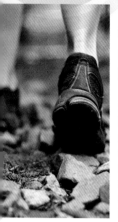

**Osteoporosis, or brittle bones, affects** an estimated one in three women and one in twelve men over the age of fifty, though many younger people are affected too. Dietary deficiencies can be a contributing factor, so it's vital to make sure you're getting the right nutrients.

Osteoporosis literally means 'porous bones'. It develops when bone-remodelling becomes unbalanced, so that not enough new bone is made to replace the old, worn-out bone that is naturally reabsorbed. As a result, bones start to thin, so the weight of carrying the upper body may lead to a vertebral fracture, while a fall can result in a hip or wrist fracture.

## Foods that can help

- **Get a good calcium intake** – this is vital throughout life. A pint (600 ml) of skimmed or semi-skimmed milk provides over 700 mg calcium. Harvard Medical School's Institute for Aging Research has found that good intakes of milk and yogurt are associated with higher bone mineral density in the hip. Other calcium-rich foods include green leafy vegetables, salmon/pilchards (tinned with bones), eggs, nuts, seeds, pulses, plus white and brown bread made from fortified flour.
- **Increase intake of vitamin D** – essential for the absorption of calcium and phosphate. Dietary sources include oily fish, liver, eggs, butter, fortified milk and fortified margarine/spreads.
- **Eat at least five servings of fruit and veg per day** for bone-friendly micronutrients such as isoflavones, carotenoids, potassium, magnesium, boron, copper, folic acid, manganese, potassium, silica, vitamin C and zinc.

## Foods to avoid

- **Avoid heavy consumption of red meat,** which is linked with early osteoporosis.
- **Cut back on caffeine:** women who drink four cups of coffee a day are three times more likely to suffer a hip fracture in later life. To offset this effect, some experts suggest obtaining an extra 40 mg calcium for every 178 ml (6 fl oz) cup of caffeinated coffee consumed.
- **Cut back on salt,** as salt increases calcium loss through your kidneys.
- **Avoid excessive alcohol intake,** which reduces absorption of calcium from your diet.
- **Avoid canned, fizzy drinks that contain phosphoric acid** – this leaches calcium from bones.

## What causes it? OSTEOPOROSIS IS LINKED WITH:

● family history ● early menopause (before age forty-five) ● loss of periods for any cause except pregnancy ● corticosteroid treatment ● little exposure to sunlight ● long-term immobility ● excess alcohol ● smoking ● intestinal malabsorption (for instance, due to coeliac disease) ● low dietary intakes of vitamin D, calcium, magnesium and phosphorus

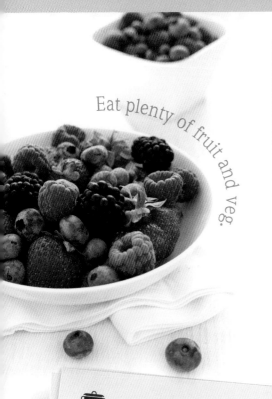

*Eat plenty of fruit and veg.*

## Osteoporosis checklist

● **Exercise regularly.** High-impact exercise (such as aerobics, racket sports, jogging) builds new bone, while, for older people, any activity (walking, gardening, climbing stairs) is useful. These activities also strengthen muscles to reduce the likelihood of a fall.

● **Don't smoke.**

● **Avoid aluminium-based antacids** – regular use for more than ten years doubles the risk of hip fracture.

● **Avoid excess stress:** stress hormones have a direct harmful effect on bone, and also reduce production of sex hormones by the adrenal glands, which provide useful top-ups in later life.

● **Consider calcium and vitamin D supplements,** which are protective.

● **Get some sun:** 15 minutes' exposure to bright sunshine, without sunscreen, can boost vitamin D levels without burning.

## 🍲 Berry Crunchy

handful of fresh mixed berries (such as raspberries, blueberries, strawberries), chopped

100 ml (14 fl oz) low-fat, low-sugar yogurt (try natural for breakfast, vanilla for dessert)

handful of flaked almonds
handful of pumpkin seeds
handful of sesame seeds

**(serves 4)**

● Divide the berries between four glasses. Spoon the yogurt over the top and sprinkle with the flaked almonds, pumpkin and sesame seeds.

# Osteoarthritis (OA)

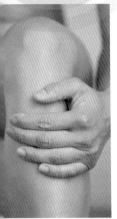

**Osteoarthritis is a progressive degeneration** of certain joints. Around one in six men and one in four women over the age of forty-five has X-ray evidence of OA within their knee joints, although only half experience pain. Foods that reduce inflammation can help to alleviate symptoms.

Osteoarthritis is associated with deteriorating quality of the cartilage lining mobile joints. It most commonly affects weight-bearing joints such as the knees, hips and lower spine, but joints used repetitively, such as the jaw, wrist and fingers, can also be affected. Articular cartilage becomes weaker, stiffer and less able to withstand compressive forces. As it cracks and flakes away, the underlying exposed bone becomes inflamed. Inflammation, loss of cartilage and joint deformity lead to stiffness and restricted movements. Walking awkwardly causes ligaments and muscles to ache.

By the age of sixty, almost 80 per cent of people show evidence of OA in at least one joint. Women are twice as likely as men to develop symptoms.

## Foods that can help

- **Consume more omega-3s:** omega-3 fatty acids are converted to substances called resolvins that 'resolve' inflammation and reduce the activity of inflammatory enzymes in the same way as aspirin. Omega-3s are found in oily fish such as mackerel, herring, salmon, trout and sardines (ideally eat two to four portions per week; *see also* page 28), wild game meat such as venison and buffalo, grass-fed beef and omega-3 enriched eggs.
- **Increase vitamin D intake,** as vitamin D protects against OA. Eat more oily fish, liver, eggs, butter and fortified milks or margarine.

## OA checklist

- **Exercise on most days** to help maintain muscle strength.
- **Exercise on even ground** and use a walking stick if necessary.
- **Avoid prolonged kneeling or squatting,** and lifting very heavy weights.
- **Use ice massage or ice packs** to help relieve joint pain.
- **Get some sun:** 15 minutes' exposure to bright sunshine (without sunscreen) can boost vitamin D levels without burning.

## What causes it? OSTEOARTHRITIS IS LINKED WITH:

- age ● family history ● gender ● occupational overuse of joints ● obesity
- sports ● trauma

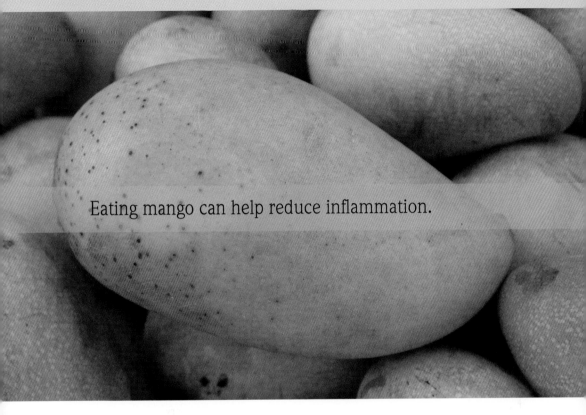

Eating mango can help reduce inflammation.

- **Eat Brazil nuts:** studies have found that those with the highest dietary intake of selenium are least likely to develop osteoarthritis, and Brazils are the richest dietary source (two Brazil nuts a day is plenty). Other sources include seafood, offal and, in some countries (such as the US and Canada), wheat flour. (In most of Europe, China and New Zealand, lack of selenium in the soil means that produce is low in this important trace nutrient.)

- **Eat the right types of fruit and veg.** Dark green leafy vegetables such as broccoli, spinach and spring greens supply antioxidant carotenoids, vitamin C, calcium and magnesium, which are beneficial for joints. Yellow/orange fruit and vegetables such as carrots, sweet potatoes, guava, mango and pumpkin are rich

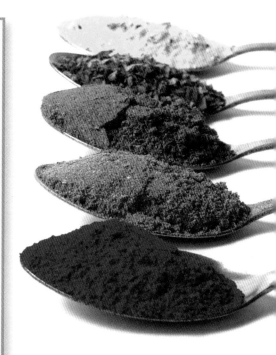

## USEFUL SUPPLEMENTS

- **A multivitamin and mineral** will help guard against nutrient deficiencies, if cutting back on food intake to lose weight
- **Omega-3 fish supplements** reduce the need for painkillers (if you eat no oily fish, you may need high-strength capsules to provide a therapeutic level of 3 g daily)
- **Vitamin D** protects against OA by improving the quality or quantity of cartilage produced by cartilage cells (look for supplements supplying vitamin D3, as these are more effective)
- **Vitamin C** helps to reduce the risk of OA progressing and knee pain developing
- **Vitamin E** to help reduce pain: one study showed that taking it daily for six weeks reduced OA pain at rest, pain on movement and the need for painkillers
- **Glucosamine sulphate** and chondroitin sulphate stimulate formation of cartilage and reduce inflammation and pain in two out of three people
- **MSM** is a source of sulphur needed for repair of joint cartilage and has been found to improve joint pain and physical functioning after twelve weeks
- **Devil's claw, ginger and rose hip** extracts contain unique compounds with a painkilling action that is similar to that of non-steroidal anti-inflammatory drugs (NSAIDs)

that inhibit the expression of inflammatory chemicals in arthritic joints and help to protect cartilage from breaking down in osteoarthritis.

sources of vitamin C and antioxidant carotenoids that can reduce inflammation in all types of arthritis.
- **Spice things up:** curry spices such as anise, chilli, cloves, cumin, fennel, ginger, mustard and turmeric have an anti-inflammatory painkilling action that may improve arthritic pain.
- **Drink more tea:** tea – especially white and green teas – contains high levels of antioxidant catechins

## Foods to avoid

- **Reduce intake of omega-6 fatty acids,** as excess dietary levels promote inflammation in the body. Eat less omega-6 vegetable oils such as safflower, grapeseed, sunflower, corn, cottonseed and soybean (replace with healthier oils such as rapeseed, olive, walnut or macadamia), less margarines based on omega-6 oils, and avoid convenience foods, fast foods and manufactured goods such us cakes, sweets and pastries.

- **Try cutting out tomatoes, peppers, chillies, aubergines and potatoes** (plants of the nightshade family) for a few weeks to see if symptoms improve, if other approaches have failed. Although controversial, sensitivity to chemicals (glycoalkaloids) found in these plants may worsen joint pain in some people (but not others).

## DID YOU KNOW?

For every 1 kg (2¼ lb) increase in weight, the overall force across your knee joints when walking or standing increases by 2–3 kg (4½–6½ lb). Losing excess weight can reduce the load exerted on weight-bearing joints as much as fourfold.

 ## Salmon Trout with Brazil Nuts

4 small salmon trout, deboned
100 g (3½ oz) Brazil nuts, chopped
4 tbsp fresh parsley, chopped
zest and juice of 1 unwaxed lemon
2 cloves garlic, crushed

freshly ground black pepper
100 g (3½ oz) Florence fennel, chopped into matchsticks

(serves 4)

- Preheat the oven to 190°C/375°F/Gas 5.
- Clean the salmon trout and remove heads, fins and tails. Stuff each deboned fish with nuts, parsley and lemon zest. Sprinkle with the lemon juice and garlic and season well with black pepper.
- Place the fennel sticks in a baking dish and arrange the salmon trout on top. Cover with foil and bake for 20–30 minutes until the flesh is just set.

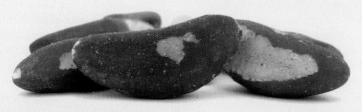

Brazils are the richest dietary source of selenium.

# Rheumatoid arthritis (RA)

**Rheumatoid arthritis affects around** 1 per cent of the population, with five times as many women affected as men. A quarter of patients develop symptoms before age thirty, but most new cases occur in the forty-to-fifty age group. Eating foods that are protective and ease joint inflammation can help.

RA is an inflammatory disease in which the synovial membranes lining some joints become thickened and inflamed, leading to redness, stiffness, swelling and pain. Inflammation gradually spreads to involve the underlying bone, which becomes worn and distorted. Usually, RA affects the smaller joints in your hands and feet, but it can also occur in the neck, wrists, knees and ankles. People with RA often feel unwell and may notice weight loss, fever and inflammation in other parts of their body such as the eyes.

Keep warm in winter.

## RA checklist

- **Avoid cold draughts** and keep as warm as possible in winter.
- **Exercise stiff hands in hot, soapy water** first thing in the morning and throughout the day.
- **Try frequent hot baths/showers;** hot or cold compresses may also be helpful.
- **Consider taking fish oils and green-lipped mussel extracts** to help relieve joint tenderness and fatigue.

## Foods that can help

- **Try going vegetarian:** eating a vegan or lactovegetarian (includes dairy products) diet improves symptoms; studies show a reduction in the number of tender and swollen joints, pain, duration of morning stiffness, grip strength and overall health assessment score after just four weeks. (If following a vegan diet, consider taking supplements supplying vitamins $B_{12}$ and D, iron and zinc.)
- **Eat your greens:** a high intake of vegetables seems to be protective, especially cruciferous vegetables

such as cabbage, broccoli, pak choi, spinach, kohlrabi and Chinese leaves.

● **Consume more olive oil:** Greek studies have found that those with greater olive oil consumption were 38 per cent less likely to develop RA.

● **Eat more fish:** more than two servings of grilled or baked fish per week has been shown to halve the risk of developing RA, compared to those eating less than one serving.

● **Get plenty of vitamin D:** a good intake is protective; sources include oily fish, fish liver oils, eggs, butter, fortified milk and supplements.

● **Eat avocado:** avocado contains antioxidant monounsaturated oils, essential fatty acids, beta-sitosterol and vitamin E that can suppress joint inflammation (avocado extracts are currently being investigated as a medical treatment for inflamed joints).

● **Get fruity:** dark blue-red pigmented fruits (such as cherries, grapes, blueberries, bilberries, blackberries, dark raspberries, elderberries) contain antioxidant anthocyanins that can reduce joint inflammation.

## Foods to avoid

● **Eat less meat:** dietary surveys show a link between RA and consumption of meat and meat products. High intakes are associated with twice the risk of low intakes.

 **Guacamole Boats**

flesh from 1 large, ripe avocado
juice of half a lemon or lime
30 ml (1 fl oz) extra virgin olive oil
freshly ground black pepper
Chinese leaves

**(serves 4)**

● Place all ingredients except the Chinese leaves into a liquidizer and blend to a paste. Season with black pepper. Spread on the Chinese leaves for a healthy snack.

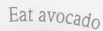

Eat avocado ...

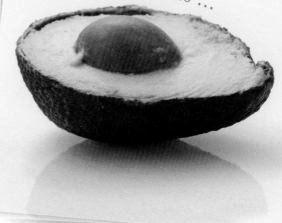

# Gout

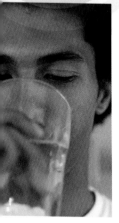

**Gout affects an estimated** one in 500 people. It's nine times more common in men than women until the time of the menopause, when incidence levels out. Dietary intervention is highly effective: one in two people manage to prevent recurrent attacks through changes in diet alone.

Gout occurs when needle-like uric acid crystals form within certain joints or soft tissues, typically at the base of the big toe. This causes excruciatingly painful arthritis with redness and swelling. Mild fever may also occur. Symptoms tend to settle within a few days, but attacks can recur several months or even years later.

Uric acid is formed from building blocks known as purines. Most purines are derived within the body from the recycling of genetic material from worn-out cells. Dietary purines account for around one-fifth of uric acid production, however, which is why dietary intervention is so beneficial.

## USEFUL SUPPLEMENTS

- **Fish oil supplements** have a useful anti-inflammatory action and do not contain purines
- **Concentrated bilberry extracts** contain antioxidants that help to lower uric acid levels
- **Devil's claw** has been found to encourage excretion of uric acid, reducing the risk of recurrent gout
- **High-dose vitamin C** mobilizes uric acid from the tissues and increases its excretion (the form known as Ester-C is best, as it's non-acidic)

**Caution:** *Avoid aspirin, as this raises uric acid levels, and avoid supplements containing more than the recommended daily amount of vitamin $B_3$ (niacin) or vitamin A, as high doses can increase uric acid levels.*

## Foods that can help

- Follow a **high-fibre, mainly vegetarian diet** with plenty of berries, fruit and vegetables, but limited animal protein.
- Eat **low-fat dairy products** (such as skimmed milk, low-fat yogurt): these appear to offer a strong protective effect, as milk proteins (casein and lactalbumin) increase the excretion of uric acid through the kidneys.
- Eat plenty of **dark blue-red fruits,** such as cherries, grapes, blueberries and bilberries: these contain antioxidants (anthocyanidins) and can lower uric acid levels and prevent gout attacks when around 250 g (9 oz) are eaten daily.

- **Have an apple a day:** apples contain malic acid, which helps to keep uric acid in solution so it is flushed from the body.
- **Drink at least 2 litres (4 pints) of water daily** to help keep uric acid in a dissolved state.

## Foods to avoid

- **Avoid purine-rich foods** such as liver, kidney, shellfish, oily fish (especially herring and sardines), game, meats and yeast extract. Some vegetables, such as asparagus, cauliflower, mushrooms, lentils and spinach, are relatively high in purines, but a recent study involving over 47,000 men suggests that moderate intakes of vegetable-based purines may not increase the risk of gout due to the beneficial antioxidants and fibre they provide.
- **Cut out sugar-sweetened soft drinks** – these have been shown to increase the risk of gout.
- **Avoid excess alcohol,** as this both increases uric acid production and reduces its excretion – especially beer, which is itself rich in purines.

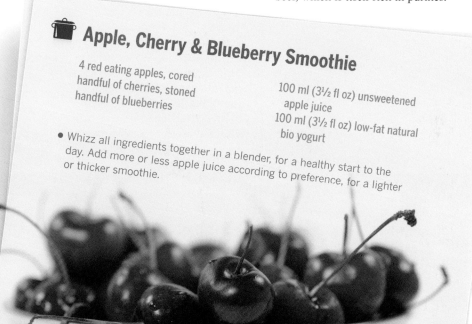

### Apple, Cherry & Blueberry Smoothie

4 red eating apples, cored
handful of cherries, stoned
handful of blueberries

100 ml (3½ fl oz) unsweetened apple juice
100 ml (3½ fl oz) low-fat natural bio yogurt

- Whizz all ingredients together in a blender, for a healthy start to the day. Add more or less apple juice according to preference, for a lighter or thicker smoothie.

# Indigestion

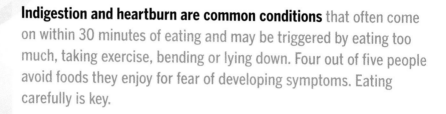

**Indigestion and heartburn are common conditions** that often come on within 30 minutes of eating and may be triggered by eating too much, taking exercise, bending or lying down. Four out of five people avoid foods they enjoy for fear of developing symptoms. Eating carefully is key.

Indigestion (or dyspepsia) is a general term used to describe any discomfort felt centrally in the upper abdomen as a result of eating. This includes feelings of distension from swallowing air, flatulence, nausea, heartburn, acidity, abdominal pain and sensations of burning. Heartburn is a more specific term referring to hot, burning sensations felt behind the chest bone, which may spread upwards toward the throat.

One of the most common causes of heartburn is acid reflux, in which stomach contents reflux up into the oesophagus (the tube connecting the mouth and stomach). This brings stomach acids and enzymes into contact with the sensitive lining of the oesophagus, and can also trigger painful spasm of muscles lining this part of the gut. In severe cases, heartburn can mimic the chest pain of a heart attack, and it has been estimated that 20 per cent of cases admitted to coronary care units may actually have gastro-oesophageal reflux disease rather than a heart problem.

## Indigestion checklist

- **Lose any excess weight.**
- **Wear loose clothing,** especially around the waist.
- **Don't smoke.**
- **Avoid aspirin and related drugs** (such as ibuprofen), which can irritate the stomach lining.
- **Try elevating the head of your bed** (prop the top two legs up on books) about 15–20 cm (6–8 in) if symptoms come on when lying down.
- **Stay calm:** stress is thought to be a major cause of indigestion – so relax and give yourself time to enjoy your food.
- **Seek medical advice** if symptoms persist or are recurrent.

## Foods that can help

Try to eat little and often throughout the day to avoid over-filling your stomach, and take care not to stoop, bend or lie down immediately after eating.

## What causes it? INDIGESTION IS LINKED WITH:

- over-indulging in rich, acidic or spicy foods • excess alcohol • smoking • being overweight • weakness of the valve between the stomach and oesophagus • hiatus hernia • anxiety/stress • acid reflux • peptic ulcers • gallbladder disease

- **Eat bland, non-acidic, easily digestible foods** such as cooked white rice, oats, scrambled eggs, ripe bananas, well-cooked green leafy vegetables, water melon, chicken broth and yogurt. Plain crackers and digestive biscuits are also worth trying.
- **Consume milk and yogurt** – these provide calcium salts that help to neutralize excess acid.
- **Try papaya:** this contains digestive enzymes that may help (for more information on digestive enzymes, *see* page 116).
- **Drink probiotic drinks or eat live bio yogurt** to maintain a high population of probiotic bacteria, which play a key role in intestinal health.

- **Drink aloe vera juice** – aloe vera is a natural antacid (do not drink during pregnancy/breastfeeding).

## Foods to avoid

- **Avoid eating large meals** (three or more courses) that are rich (for instance, including cream sauces) or 'heavy' (including pastries, gateaux or cheesecake).
- **Steer clear of acidic fruit juices, coffee and alcohol** as much as possible, as these are the commonest culprits for triggering symptoms.
- **Avoid late-night eating.**
- **Don't drink fluids with meals,** as these dilute digestive juices (although water or milk are desirable if you have reflux).

 ## Soothing Banana Rice Pudding

200 g (7 oz) cooked white rice
2 ripe bananas, mashed
300 ml (10 fl oz) low-fat vanilla
bio yogurt

sprinkle of cinnamon

(serves 4)

- Combine all the ingredients. Serve cold or warmed through (don't overheat), with an extra sprinkle of cinnamon on top.

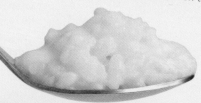

# Bloating

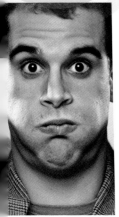

**Although bloating is commonly linked with** over-indulgence or eating a rich, fatty diet, it can also occur after eating relatively little in those with functional disorders of the gut. Ensuring adequate intake of digestive enzymes can help.

Your salivary glands, stomach, small intestines, liver and pancreas produce a variety of digestive enzymes needed to process your food properly. These include proteases, which break down dietary proteins, amylases, which digest carbohydrates, and lipases, which break down dietary fats. As you get older, you tend to produce less intestinal enzymes and less stomach acid, which can lead to a number of health problems, from bloating, wind and heartburn to irritable bowel syndrome and malabsorption.

## Bloating checklist

- **Eat slowly,** chewing each mouthful well.
- **Avoid fizzy drinks, drinking through a straw, chewing gum and sucking on boiled sweets** – these increase air-swallowing and gassiness.
- **Seek medical advice** if symptoms last more than two weeks.

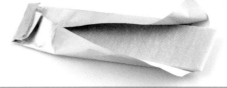

## Foods that can help

- **Enjoy tropical fruit:** digestive enzymes are found in many plant foods, especially pineapples, kiwi and papaya.
- **Consume more fruit, vegetables, salads and juices** – these contain potassium, which helps to flush excess sodium from the body to reduce fluid retention.
- **Increase magnesium intake:** magnesium plays an important role in salt and fluid balance; food sources include fish, nuts, seeds, soybeans, wholegrains and dark green leafy vegetables.
- **Drink peppermint, ginger or fennel tea** – these can help to reduce bloating.
- **Eat live bio yogurt** or other sources of probiotic digestive bacteria.

DIGESTIVE ENZYME SUPPLEMENTS
These are available from health food stores, but do check the labels, as those with the highest number of 'activity units' are the most effective. If you feel bloated after eating carbohydrate, try carbohydrate-digesting enzymes such as amylase and cellulase. If

- eating too much • eating too quickly • lack of digestive enzymes • reduced bile output
- swallowing air • fluid retention • reduced function or enlargement of an internal organ
- physical obstructions of the gut

milk causes a problem, consider milk-digesting enzymes containing bromelain (from pineapples), papain (from papaya), lipase and lactase. If you are gluten-intolerant, a product supplying gluten protease, cellulase and amylase can help.

To improve general digestion, select a mixed digestive enzyme supplement containing lipase (digests fats), amylase (digests carbohydrates), protease (digests protein), lactase (digests milk sugar) and cellulase (digests cellulose).

## Foods to avoid

- **Cut back on salty foods and 'windy' foods** such as beans, lentils and onions.
- **Switch to lactose-free dairy products** if you have a lactose intolerance.

### OTHER USEFUL SUPPLEMENTS

- **Dandelion** is a natural herbal diuretic widely used to flush excess fluid from the body
- **Globe artichoke** extracts significantly boost bile production and can quickly relieve bloating due to poor bile output, especially if symptoms are linked with fatty foods, drinking alcohol or if your gallbladder has been removed

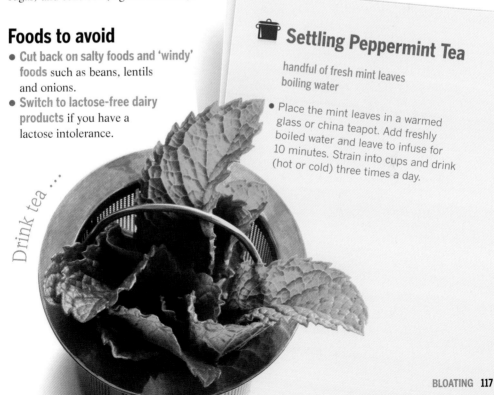

### 🍲 Settling Peppermint Tea

handful of fresh mint leaves
boiling water

- Place the mint leaves in a warmed glass or china teapot. Add freshly boiled water and leave to infuse for 10 minutes. Strain into cups and drink (hot or cold) three times a day.

Drink tea ...

# Gallstones

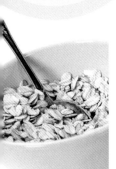

**Gallstones are four times more common** in women than in men, and as many as one in five women develop gallstones at some time in their life. Getting your daily oats and eating a low-fat, high-fibre diet could be the key to combating this common condition.

Gallstones form in the gallbladder, a pouch-like organ that stores bile – a green-yellow, detergent-like substance made in the liver that digests dietary fats into small globules so they're easier to absorb. Gallstones develop when ingredients dissolved in bile precipitate out to form solids. Most gallstones are made of cholesterol, although some contain high amounts of bile pigments or calcium salts.

Gallstones tend to be round or oval in shape, and range in size from 1 to 25 mm (up to 1 in) across. Some people develop one large stone, while others harbour up to 200 or more tiny grit-like stones. Only one in five people who have gallstones will go on to develop symptoms of colicky, upper abdominal pain, which can be quite severe.

## Foods that can help

- **Follow a low-fat, high-fibre diet,** as dietary fat triggers contraction of the gallbladder, which may push a gallstone into the mouth of the bile duct to cause pain. (NOTE: Some fats have a beneficial effect on cholesterol balance, however, such as olive, rapeseed and nut oils, which may help to prevent gallstones.)
- **Eat oily fish two or three times a week,** as omega-3 fish oils are beneficial.
- **Opt for oatmeal:** plants rich in soluble fibre such as pectins (found in apples, carrots, apricots) and gums (found in oat bran and beans) bind cholesterol and bile salts to reduce their re-absorption. In fact, eating one bowl of oatmeal a day can reduce your 'bad' LDL- cholesterol level by 8–23 percent. Have porridge or unsweetened oatmeal-based muesli for breakfast, mix rolled oats into yogurts, and eat oatcakes as a snack.

## Gallstone checklist

- **Limit alcohol intake** to within recommended healthy levels.
- **Lose any excess fat** to maintain a healthy body weight.
- **Eat at least five servings of fruit, vegetables and salad foods** every day.

## What causes it? GALLSTONES ARE LINKED WITH:

- female gender • family history • being overweight • high-fat diet • having taken the oral contraceptive pill or HRT

- **Use fresh young dandelion leaves in salads** – a traditional herbal remedy for gallstones.
- **Drink plenty of fluids** – especially water or herbal teas – to keep well hydrated and prevent sludging of bile.

### USEFUL SUPPLEMENTS

- **Milk thistle extracts** have beneficial effects on the composition of bile
- **Vitamin C supplements** help to prevent cholesterol from solidifying out of bile to form stones

 ## Oat, Apple & Carrot Muffins

160 g (5½ oz) rolled oats
30 g (1 oz) wholewheat flour
2 tsp baking powder
½ tsp salt
1 tsp cinnamon
1 tsp ground ginger
2 omega-3 enriched eggs

100 g (3½ oz) dark brown sugar
120 ml (4 fl oz) olive oil
100 g (3½ oz) carrots, grated
1 red apple, cored and grated
handful dried apricots, finely chopped

(makes 12)

- Preheat the oven to 200°C/400°F/Gas 6.
- Using a food processor, pulverize the oats for 1 minute. Transfer to a bowl, add the flour, baking powder, salt, cinnamon and ginger and mix together.
- In a separate bowl, beat the eggs until fluffy, then beat in the sugar and oil. Add the pre-mixed dry ingredients and fold in. When combined, fold in the carrots, apple and apricots.
- Pile into 12 muffin cups. Bake for 20–25 minutes until a cocktail stick or skewer comes out clean.

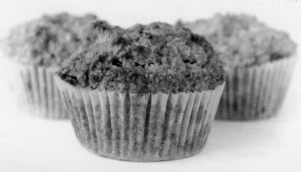

# Constipation & diverticular disease

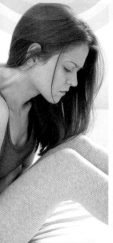

**Constipation affects us all** at some time, while ongoing problems (chronic constipation) affect one in eight of the general population. Eating a high-fibre diet, with plenty of fluids, gives you the best chance of combating this often painful condition.

Chronic constipation is diagnosed when someone (who does not have irritable bowel syndrome) experiences at least two of the following for three months: less than three bowel movements per week, straining, lumpy/hard stools, sensation of anorectal obstruction, sensation of incomplete defecation and/or requires manual assistance to pass a motion.

Those most commonly affected are young children, the elderly, people with irritable bowel syndrome and women who are pregnant (due to the smooth-muscle-relaxing effects of progesterone hormone). Constipation and straining can lead to haemorrhoids and to diverticular disease, in which increased pressure causes the lining of the colon to rupture through its overlying muscle. This produces small out-pouchings (diverticulae) that make constipation worse (by interfering with muscle contraction) and which may become infected, inflamed and painful (diverticulitis). Diverticular disease affects an estimated one in three people between the ages of fifty and sixty, and becomes increasingly common above this age.

## Foods that can help

Fibre aids the digestion and absorption of foods, promotes a healthy bacterial balance and provides important bulk to stimulate peristalsis – the muscular, wave-like motion that transports

## USEFUL SUPPLEMENTS

- **Natural bulking agents** (bran, psyllium/ ispaghula, sterculia) taken with plenty of water help to increase frequency of bowel movements
- **Magnesium supplements** (tablets, or as Epsom salts dissolved in warm water) are an effective laxative – take at night to gain benefit the following morning
- **Cold pressed oils** such as virgin olive oil, safflower, walnut or sesame may help – take 1–2 tablespoons at night
- **Molasses** is an effective and harmless laxative – take 1–2 teaspoons daily
- **Probiotic supplements** (such as Lactobacilli, Bifidobacteria) help to maintain optimum bowel function
- **Aloe vera juice** has a useful cleansing and soothing action on the intestines (do not take during pregnancy or breastfeeding)

## What causes it? CONSTIPATION IS LINKED WITH:

- age • pregnancy • low-fibre diet • dehydration • lack of exercise • poor pelvic muscle tone
- irritable bowel syndrome • hernia • medication (especially opiate pain-killers) • underactive thyroid • abdominal tumours (such as a large ovarian cyst, fibroids) • bowel obstruction

### DID YOU KNOW?

**There may be** some truth in the saying that constipation is associated with 'a change of water'. If you come from a hard water area, with a high percentage of dissolved calcium and magnesium, you may adapt less well to soft water areas where your intake of these minerals (needed for muscle contraction) may be reduced.

### DRUGS THAT CAN CAUSE CONSTIPATION

- Painkillers (especially codeine phosphate)
- Antacids (especially aluminium-based ones)
- Tricyclic antidepressants (such as amitriptyline)
- Calcium antagonists (such as nifedipine)
- Iron preparations
- Steroids
- Overuse of laxatives (the bowel becomes less responsive to their action)

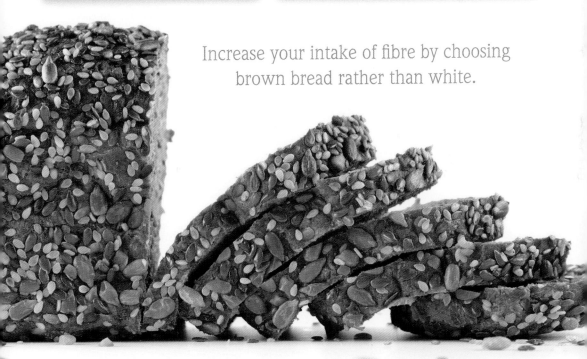

Increase your intake of fibre by choosing brown bread rather than white.

## Constipation checklist

- **Take regular exercise** (such as walking, swimming or cycling): this strengthens abdominal muscles and encourages bowel activity.
- **Apply hot and cold compresses** to your abdomen and follow with an aromatherapy massage: gently massage the abdomen in a clockwise direction, starting on the lower left side, with diluted oils of ginger, lemon, sandalwood, mandarin, orange, grapefruit or neroli (blend three or four together if you wish).
- **Insert a glycerol suppository** to help ease motions and reduce straining. Straining can also be reduced by leaning forwards from the hips when opening your bowels.
- **Use a 'squatty potty'** (this raises your feet when going to the toilet, and improves your position for optimum elimination).
- **Seek medical advice** if constipation lasts more than five days, or is associated with abdominal pain, vomiting or passing blood/mucus.

digested food through the intestines. It's therefore important to make sure you're getting enough in your diet.

### SOURCES OF FIBRE

Increase fibre intake slowly, so you don't develop wind and bloating from an initial fibre overload. Select brown rather than white bread, brown rice, wholewheat pasta, wholegrain cereals, oats, whole rye, buckwheat, millet, and unsweetened wholegrain breakfast cereals such as muesli or porridge. In addition:

- **Eat more** nuts, figs, dates, apricots, prunes, peas, beans, salads and other fresh fruit and vegetables; try soaking 5–6 prunes in water or cold tea overnight and eat for breakfast with bio yogurt.

Figs are an excellent source of dietary fibre.

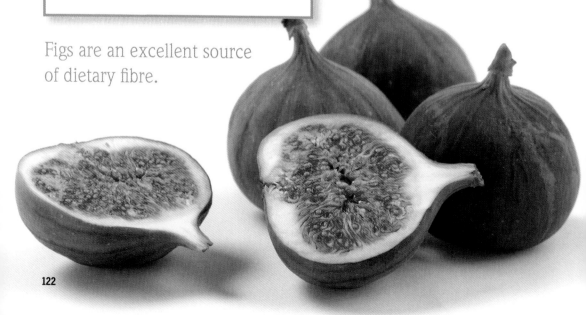

## DID YOU KNOW?

**Bowel bacteria** adapt to the types of fibre you eat. If you're taking fibre supplements, vary these every month or so, before bacterial enzymes adapt to break them down more readily.

# Oaty, banana date cookies

125 g (4½ oz) rolled oats
125 g (4½ oz) dates, chopped (or chopped figs, apricots, raisins, sultanas)
75 g (3 oz) shredded coconut
50 g (2 oz) ground almonds
40 g (1½ oz) mixed chopped nuts
½ tsp salt
1 tsp cinnamon
½ tsp allspice
3 large, ripe bananas, mashed
60 ml (2 fl oz) hempseed or rapeseed oil
1 tsp vanilla extract

**(makes 12)**

- Preheat the oven to 175°C/350°F/Gas 4 and line a baking sheet with parchment paper.
- Combine all dry ingredients (including dried fruit) and mix well, ensuring the fruit doesn't clump together.
- In another bowl, combine the mashed banana, oil and vanilla extract. Add the dry ingredients and stir until well combined.
- Place a cooking ring/pastry cutter on the baking sheet and press spoonfuls of the mix into it, according to your preferred biscuit thickness. Remove the cutter and repeat. Bake for 20 minutes, or until edges are golden brown. Leave to cool slightly on the baking sheet, before transferring to a cooling rack.

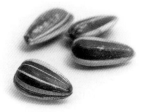

- **Add seeds** (such as sunflower, pumpkin, fenugreek, fennel and linseed) to salads and yogurt for extra roughage.
- **Drink plenty of fluids** – a good fluid intake is vital. Try freshly squeezed fruit juice (such as mango and apple), carrot juice and water. Probiotic drinks and bio yogurt will ensure a healthy balance of digestive bacteria.

## Foods to avoid

- **Steer clear of processed 'white' versions of flour, bread, pasta and rice**, as these have had their beneficial fibre stripped out.

# Food allergy & intolerance

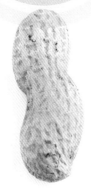

**Official figures suggest that** 2 per cent of adults and up to 8 per cent of children have a classic, potentially life-threatening food allergy, while as many as one in three people suffer from food intolerance. Identifying trigger foods is key in preventing the onset of symptoms.

Foods that trigger a classic allergic reaction involve a type of antibody known as IgE. This interacts with immune cells in the skin, intestines and respiratory tract to cause the release of powerful chemicals, such as histamine. In some people, this causes a severe, life-threatening anaphylactic reaction, with falling blood pressure, constriction of airways, facial/tongue swelling and collapse. These symptoms tend to come on quickly, usually within minutes of exposure.

In contrast, symptoms linked with food intolerances are usually delayed, coming on many hours or even days after the culprit food was eaten. Delayed immune responses to food are thought to result from other immune mechanisms that may involve other classes of antibody (such as IgG), immune-complexes and abnormal immune cell responses. While intolerance is a less serious condition than classic food allergy, symptoms can nonetheless be extremely unpleasant, ranging from a running nose, catarrh and fatigue to irritable bowel syndrome, joint pain, headache and inflammatory problems such as asthma, eczema, psoriasis, Crohn's disease or ulcerative colitis.

## COMMON ALLERGY TRIGGERS

Foods that can trigger an IgE mediated 'classic' food allergy include:

- Eggs
- Cow's milk
- Peanuts
- Tree nuts
- Shellfish
- Fin fish
- Wheat
- Soy
- Beef
- Chicken
- Citrus fruits
- Tomatoes

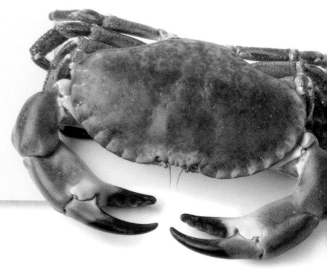

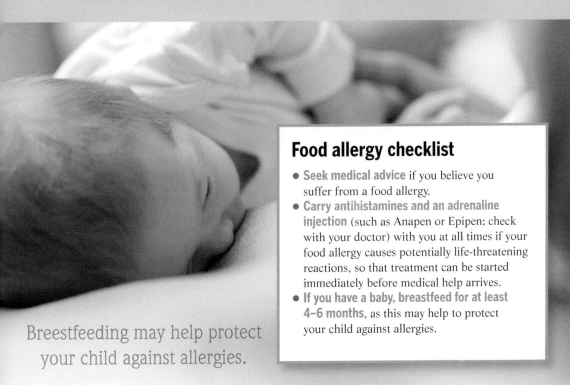

## What causes it? FOOD ALLERGIES & INTOLERANCES ARE LINKED WITH:

- family history ● early weaning ● environmental factors ● antibiotics ● possibly modern over-cleanliness, which reduces immune-priming by intestinal worms and bacteria

Breestfeeding may help protect
your child against allergies.

## Food allergy checklist

- **Seek medical advice** if you believe you suffer from a food allergy.
- **Carry antihistamines and an adrenaline injection** (such as Anapen or Epipen; check with your doctor) with you at all times if your food allergy causes potentially life-threatening reactions, so that treatment can be started immediately before medical help arrives.
- **If you have a baby, breastfeed for at least 4–6 months**, as this may help to protect your child against allergies.

Some of the more defined food intolerances include:

- **lactose intolerance** – the inability to digest lactose sugar in milk, causing bloating, abdominal pain and diarrhoea in those not producing sufficient amounts of the enzyme lactase
- **gluten intolerance** – an autoimmune condition in which sensitivity to a protein (gliadin) found in wheat and some other cereals causes bloating, abdominal pain, bulky stools and weight loss (*see* coeliac disease, page 128)
- **food hypersensitivity**, in which a widespread, itchy rash (urticaria), eczema, asthma, vomiting, abdominal pains or diarrhoea can occur through eating certain foods. In some cases, these are due to high levels of naturally occurring histamine found in foods such as tuna (scrombroid poisoning), strawberries, fermented foods, tomatoes, cheese, aubergine or citrus fruits

*Eggs are a common food-allergy trigger.*

## DID YOU KNOW?

**Food intolerance tests** that identify raised levels of IgG antibodies against particular foods may help to identify foods to which you are intolerant, without having to follow a time-consuming elimination and challenge diet.

- **drug-like reactions**, in which chemicals such as monosodium glutamate, sulphites, salicylates, benzoates, tartrazine and tyramine present in certain foods can trigger symptoms such as asthma or migraine

A popular theory suggests that over-cleanliness and excessive use of antibiotics has caused our T-helper immune cells to move away from anti-infective reactions towards allergic-type sensitivity reactions.

## Foods that can help

The diagnosis of food sensitivity is traditionally made when symptoms disappear during an elimination diet and reappear when the suspected food is reintroduced – even in hidden form. There are several degrees of exclusion diet ranging from:

- **simple exclusion** – elimination of a single food such as eggs
- **multiple exclusion** – elimination of several foods that have been linked with a particular problem

- **restriction diet** – which consists of eating very few foods: for example, nothing but a single meat (such as lamb, turkey, wild game), a single source of carbohydrate (such as rice, tapioca), a single fruit (such as pears, pear juice, cranberries), selected vegetables (such as squash, carrots, parsnips, lettuce, lentils, split peas) and drinking spring, mineral or distilled water

After following the elimination diet until symptoms have disappeared (commonly between ten and twenty-one days), the eliminated foods are reintroduced one by one, usually at three- or four-day intervals, to see which triggers a recurrence. You will need to keep a careful food and symptom diary during this time, to help recognize which particular foods – if any – are triggering your symptoms. If an adverse reaction occurs, continue to avoid the test food and wait 48 hours after all symptoms have improved before testing another food.

If your symptoms are not significantly improved by following a restricted diet, it's important to return to eating a normal diet, and to eating as wide a range of foods as possible, to guard against nutrient deficiencies. If you are able to identify a small number of foods that provoke your symptoms, however, these can usually be avoided without affecting your overall nutrition.

## Foods to avoid

Avoid any food that you recognize as being associated with your symptoms. Eight foods are responsible for 90 per cent of all food allergies. These are eggs, peanuts, milk, wheat, soy, tree nuts (for example walnuts, Brazils and cashews), fish and shellfish. Foods that

are increasingly being associated with allergy include kiwi, papaya, sesame, rapeseed, poppy seeds and psyllium, although the risk is low.

### USEFUL SUPPLEMENTS

- **Probiotic bacteria** may reduce the development of allergic conditions such as eczema by stimulating the production of antibodies rather than allergic reactions. As a result, probiotics appear to reduce the development of eczema during at least the first four years of life. Infants should only receive probiotic supplements specifically designed for their age group, under medical supervision. It may be better to stimulate growth of their own natural probiotic bacteria through the use of prebiotics, which are now added to some baby milk formulas.

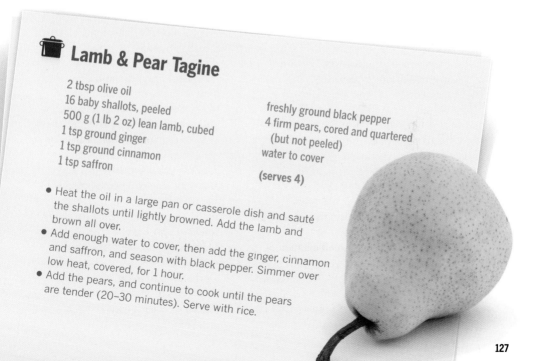

## Lamb & Pear Tagine

2 tbsp olive oil
16 baby shallots, peeled
500 g (1 lb 2 oz) lean lamb, cubed
1 tsp ground ginger
1 tsp ground cinnamon
1 tsp saffron

freshly ground black pepper
4 firm pears, cored and quartered
(but not peeled)
water to cover

(serves 4)

- Heat the oil in a large pan or casserole dish and sauté the shallots until lightly browned. Add the lamb and brown all over.
- Add enough water to cover, then add the ginger, cinnamon and saffron, and season with black pepper. Simmer over low heat, covered, for 1 hour.
- Add the pears, and continue to cook until the pears are tender (20–30 minutes). Serve with rice.

# Coeliac disease

## DID YOU KNOW?

Glutens are the proteins that give bread dough its elasticity.

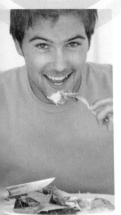

**Also known as gluten-sensitive enteropathy**, coeliac disease affects an estimated one in 100 people, although for every person who knows they have the condition, another seven remain undiagnosed. A gluten-free diet is the only way to combat this increasingly prevalent condition.

Coeliac disease is an autoimmune inflammatory disease of the small intestine. It's caused by a reaction to gliadin, a type of gluten protein found in wheat. In people with coeliac disease, gliadin triggers an immune reaction, with the production of anti-endomysial antibodies that damage the lining of the small intestine. This causes a characteristic flattening of the inner surface of the lower jejunum, which interferes with nutrient absorption. Coeliac disease leads to symptoms such as bloating, wind, abdominal pain, bulky stools, poor absorption of nutrients and weight loss unless gluten is excluded from the diet.

When eating gluten affects other parts of the body, it's referred to as non-coeliac gluten sensitivity (NCGS). Less is known about NCGS, but it is estimated to affect at least one in ten people, with symptoms that may include tiredness, recurrent mouth ulcers, skin rashes, headache and joint pain.

Someone who is sensitive to the wheat gliadin form of gluten is often sensitive to glutens found in other cereals, too, because of the similar amino acid chains they contain. It is relatively common for people with coeliac disease to react to rye and

## Coeliac checklist

- **See your doctor for a blood test** if you think you could have gluten sensitivity, to confirm whether or not you are affected.
- **Maintain a strict gluten-free diet for life.**
- **Check food labels carefully** to look for hidden gluten.
- **Talk to your pharmacist,** if you have concerns about the contents of any medication (wheat starch is sometimes added to medicines, but it is of pharmaceutical quality and considered gluten-free).
- **Use cosmetics labelled as gluten-free,** if bowel or skin symptoms persist despite a gluten-free diet (although gluten is not absorbed through the skin, when used in lipstick or foundation small amounts may be ingested).

## What causes it? COELIAC DISEASE IS LINKED WITH:

• family history • previous bowel infection (for example, with rotavirus) • early weaning • other autoimmune conditions such as type 1 diabetes • ulcerative colitis • autoimmune thyroid disease

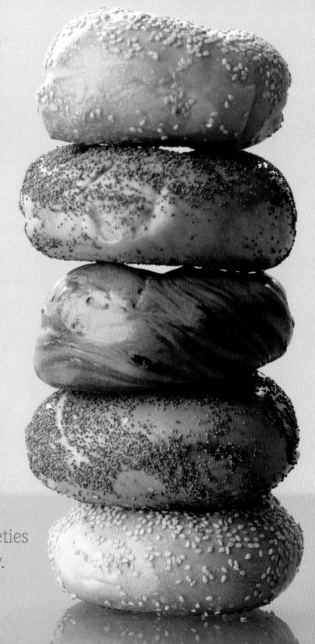

| GRAIN | FORM OF GLUTEN |
|-------|----------------|
| Wheat | gliadin |
| Rye | secalin |
| Barley | hordein |
| Oats | avenin |
| Maize | zein |

barley, but they are less likely to react to the gluten in oats. Maize usually causes no problem.

## Foods that can help

If your doctor has confirmed coeliac disease via a blood test, following a strict gluten/gliadin-free diet for life allows the inflammatory changes in your intestinal lining to resolve, so your intestines regain their normal function. A gluten-free diet allows you to eat a wide variety of nutritious foods, including:

• fruit, vegetables and salad foods
• beans, peas, lentils
• nuts and seeds
• unprocessed meat, poultry or offal
• plain (uncoated) fish
• eggs, cheese, milk, yogurts
  (except muesli yogurt)

Look for gluten-free varieties
of the foods you enjoy.

- rice, tapioca, sago, arrowroot, buckwheat (which, despite its name, is not related to wheat), millet, hempseed, teff and amaranth (*see* below), maize, corn and cornflour
- gluten-free bread, crispbread, biscuits, cakes, breakfast cereals and pasta
- gluten-free flour, soya flour, potato flour, pea flour, rice flour, gram flour
- sugar, jam, marmalade, honey, jelly
- herbs, spices, mustard, vinegar, salt, pepper
- milk, cream, butter, margarine and oils
- tea, coffee, fruit juice
- wine, non-barley beer, spirits

Teff is an ancient, gluten-free grain available in brown and white versions, both of which are wholegrain, as the kernel is too small to mill easily. Teff supplies more fibre-rich bran and nutritious germ than any other grain, and has a high mineral content including seventeen times more calcium than wheat or barley. Teff flour can be cooked as porridge, used as a wheat flour substitute in bread, pancakes, muffins, pasta and cakes, or made into 'teff polenta'. Amaranth is another highly nutritious gluten-free grain that can be used for all kinds of cooking and baking.

## Foods to avoid

Avoid any food labelled as containing wheat, gluten or gliadin (wheat is often present in products such as soups, stock cubes and dessert mixes). Avoid foods containing flour starch, wheat flour, wheat starch, food starch, edible

Try cooking with gluten-free flour, soya flour or potato flour instead ...

## DID YOU KNOW?

**Intolerance to** other proteins found in wheat (not gliadin) can cause symptoms that resemble irritable bowel syndrome. This is not classed as coeliac disease, as no anti-endomysial antibodies are produced.

starch, modified starch, gelatinized starch, vegetable starch, cereal filler, cereal binder, cereal protein, malt, rye, hydrolysed vegetable protein, Kamut, natural flavouring, soy sauce, gum, triticale, spelt, rusk or barley *unless they are declared gluten-free* Wheat can be processed to render it gluten-free by washing the gluten out of flour.

## USEFUL SUPPLEMENTS

- **A multivitamin and mineral** will guard against nutritional deficiencies (check it is gluten-free)
- **Aloe vera gel** has a soothing effect on the bowel; select products declared aloin-free to avoid a laxative action (avoid if pregnant or breastfeeding)

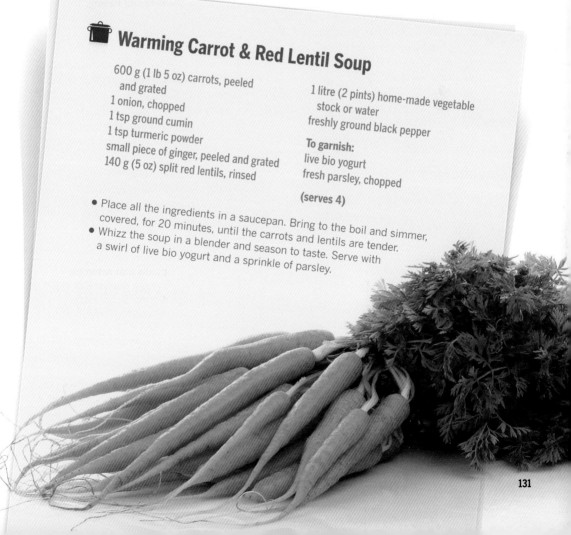

# Warming Carrot & Red Lentil Soup

600 g (1 lb 5 oz) carrots, peeled and grated
1 onion, chopped
1 tsp ground cumin
1 tsp turmeric powder
small piece of ginger, peeled and grated
140 g (5 oz) split red lentils, rinsed

1 litre (2 pints) home-made vegetable stock or water
freshly ground black pepper

**To garnish:**
live bio yogurt
fresh parsley, chopped

(serves 4)

- Place all the ingredients in a saucepan. Bring to the boil and simmer, covered, for 20 minutes, until the carrots and lentils are tender.
- Whizz the soup in a blender and season to taste. Serve with a swirl of live bio yogurt and a sprinkle of parsley.

# Irritable bowel syndrome (IBS)

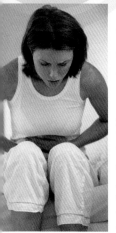

**IBS is the most common condition** to affect the gut. At least a third of us are affected at some time during our lives, and men and women are thought to be equally susceptible (though men are less likely to consult their doctor). Adjusting your diet can alleviate symptoms.

IBS is a functional condition of the gut in which contraction of muscle in the bowel wall leads to intermittent pain, bloating (with or without distension), diarrhoea and/or constipation. According to specified criteria for diagnosing irritable bowel syndrome, there must be recurrent abdominal pain or discomfort for at least three days per month in the preceding three months (with onset at least six months previously), associated with two or more of the following:

- improvement with defecation
- onset associated with change in frequency of stool
- onset associated with change in form (appearance) of stool

While IBS can affect anyone at any age, symptoms most commonly start between the ages of thirty and forty, and recent studies have suggested that more people are affected in the forty-five to sixty-five age range than in younger age groups.

## IBS checklist

- **Seek medical advice** if you think you could have IBS, especially if you are aged fifty or over at onset, have night-time symptoms, rectal bleeding, weight loss, exhaustion, recent antibiotic use or a significant family history of bowel cancer.
- **Avoid cigarette smoke** – nicotine receptors in the gut increase bowel spasm.
- **Avoid obvious causes of stress,** as stress promotes diarrhoea.
- **Take regular exercise,** as this helps to relieve bloating, distension and pain.
- **Don't rush your meals:** allow yourself plenty of time to eat, so you don't bolt down your food and swallow excessive amounts of air.

## Foods that can help

- **Select wholefoods** that are as unprocessed as possible.
- **Eat more fibre:** fibre is important to improve both diarrhoea (by absorbing fluid) and constipation (by providing bulk). Increase your fibre intake slowly, and drink plenty of fluids. Try bran, figs, apricots, prunes, peas or beans, but if these bring on your symptoms (as they do for some

people) try bananas, berries and oats, which are usually better tolerated.

● **Increase intake of complex, unrefined carbohydrates.** If your symptoms aren't made worse by wheat, go for wholegrain bread, wholemeal pasta, brown rice and unsweetened wholegrain breakfast cereals such as muesli or porridge. Alternatives to wheat include buckwheat (despite its name, it's a gluten-free member of the rhubarb family), hempseed, brown rice, red rice (Camargue or Bhutan), wild rice (a grass seed), corn, soy, amaranth and teff (*see also* coeliac disease, page 130), quinoa, gram/chickpea flour, millet and tapioca.

● **Help yourself to herbs:** a number of herbs and spices can relieve bowel spasm and reduce wind, such as aniseed, camomile, lemon balm, clove, dill, fennel, black pepper, marjoram, parsley, peppermint, rosemary and spearmint. Cook with them or use them fresh as a garnish (fresh is better than dried), or enjoy them as soothing herbal teas.

● **Eat more fish,** especially oily fish, as people with IBS often have low intakes of essential fatty acids.

● **Consume more live bio yogurt** to increase the levels of beneficial bacteria in your gut.

Eating several small meals, spread throughout the day, may be easier to digest than three larger meals, but if your lifestyle makes this tricky, then do your best to follow the old adage: breakfast like a king, lunch like a lord and dine like a pauper.

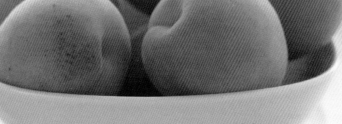

Apricots are a good source of fibre.

# Foods to avoid

Many people find benefit from a diet that is free from wheat, gluten, lactose, yeast and artificial sweeteners. The Addenbrooke's exclusion diet eliminates the foods most commonly associated with IBS symptoms, as shown in the table below:

After following this exclusion diet for two or three weeks, start reintroducing foods you're particularly fond of (one new food every three or four days). Foods that you might want to reintroduce, one at a time, include potatoes, milk, yogurt, white wine, tea, coffee, cheese, citrus fruits, butter, onions, eggs, chocolate, sweetcorn and wheat. If the new food is well tolerated, you can continue

| FOODS YOU CAN EAT | FOODS YOU SHOULD AVOID |
| --- | --- |
| Meat | All cereals except rice |
| Fish | All dairy products |
| All fruit except citrus | Eggs |
| Soy products | Yeast |
| All vegetables except potatoes, sweetcorn and onions | Caffeine |

Some herbs can help to relieve bowel spasm and reduce wind.

to keep this food in your diet. If symptoms worsen, however, that food should be avoided until you feel willing to try it again. If symptoms persistently worsen when eating that particular food – and improve when avoiding it – you should consider eliminating it from your diet long-term. (Do not follow an elimination diet for longer than two weeks without professional dietary advice.)

As with food allergies (*see* page 124) and Crohn's disease (*see* page 140), food intolerance tests that identify raised levels of IgG antibodies against particular foods may help to identify foods you have an intolerance for, without having to follow an elimination diet. Talk to a registered nutritionist to find out more.

## USEFUL SUPPLEMENTS

- **Peppermint oil** is one of the most effective treatments for IBS; trials have shown it to be more effective than either fibre or antispasmodic drugs. On average, 75 per cent of people with IBS who take peppermint oil experience a greater than 50 per cent reduction in symptoms
- **Probiotic supplements** often improve symptoms of IBS: one study showed a 75 per cent improvement in symptoms, increasing to 90 per cent when probiotic bacteria and drug treatment (mebeverine) were taken together
- **Globe artichoke supplements** help to improve symptoms; according to one study, an overall reduction in IBS symptoms of 71 per cent was achieved within an average of ten days
- **Psyllium fibre** is a well-tolerated fibre supplement
- **Aloe vera juice** has a soothing effect on the bowel – select products declared aloin-free to avoid a laxative effect (avoid if pregnant or breastfeeding)

 **Hempseed, Apricot & Date Bites**

400 g (14 oz) dried apricots, chopped
200 g (7 oz) dates, chopped
160 g (5½ oz) shelled hempseeds
zest and juice of 1 large lemon

1 tsp ground nutmeg
1 tsp ground cinnamon
1 tsp gluten-free vanilla extract

(makes 24)

- Pulse all the ingredients in a food processor to form a chunky paste, then transfer to a small, parchment-lined baking dish or tin (about 20 x 20 cm/ 8 x 8 in) and press down to an even thickness.
- Cover and chill for 1–2 hours, until firm. Cut into bite-sized squares to serve.

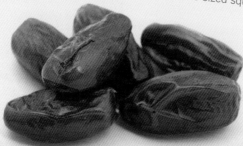

# Ulcerative colitis

**This inflammatory disease of the bowel** affects around one in 1,000 people and is most common in those aged between twenty and forty. Three out of five people affected are female. Foods containing sulphites appear to be common triggers, and may worsen symptoms.

Ulcerative colitis is associated with inflammation and ulceration of the colon lining (large bowel). The main symptom is blood-stained diarrhoea, which may also contain pus and mucus. In severe attacks, fever, abdominal pain and feelings of being quite unwell can also occur. Attacks tend to come on every few months, although some people experience infrequent symptoms, while, for others, symptoms are continuous.

Researchers have compared the food and drink consumed by people who suffer from ulcerative colitis with the visual appearance of the bowel lining. This has pinpointed the dietary components most likely to be associated with active symptoms, as shown in the table opposite:

15 minutes of sensible sun exposure helps to make vitamin D.

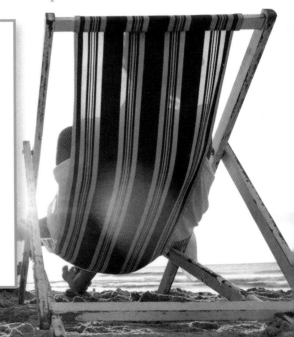

## Ulcerative colitis checklist

- **Enjoy sensible sun exposure** to make vitamin D (no more than 15 minutes without sunscreen, to avoid burning), and take vitamin D supplements.
- **Consult a dietician or medical nutritionist for supervision** if following a restrictive diet (such as one that is gluten-free), to ensure your nutritional needs are being met.
- **Avoid stress:** people with ulcerative colitis who experience a stressful life event, or persistent (chronic) stress, are more likely to have a relapse of their symptoms than those who are not stressed.

## What causes it? ULCERATIVE COLITIS IS LINKED WITH:

- family history • abnormal bowel fermentation • possibly poor gut blood supply
- abnormal immune responses

| FOODS LINKED WITH ACTIVE ULCERATIVE COLITIS | FOODS NOT ASSOCIATED WITH ULCERATIVE COLITIS |
|---|---|
| Burgers, sausages and other preserved meats (except organic non-sulphited products) | Pork, bacon |
| | Beef, beef products |
| Beer (except German beer, which is sulphite-free), lager | Fish |
| | Raw apples, pears, bananas, citrus fruits, melon |
| Red and white wine | Milk, yogurt, cheese |
| Sulphite-containing soft drinks, such as fruit squash made from concentrates | Soup (home-made, not tinned or dried) |
| Coffee (except decaffeinated brands) | Breakfast cereals |
| Prawns, scampi, shellfish (sulphited) | Lettuce, tomatoes, potatoes, peas, beans |
| Dried fruit and vegetables (sulphited) | |
| Processed fruit pies and fruit cakes | |
| Foods containing sulphites (see list of sulphite additives overleaf) | |
| Foods containing the sulphur-rich seaweed carrageenan (a gelling/thickening agent extracted from Irish Moss, identified by E-number E407) | |

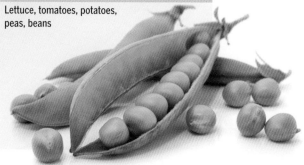

## Foods that can help

Some varieties of Bifidophilus probiotic bacteria (Bifidobacterium and Acidophilus) have shown benefits in preventing relapses and maintaining remission. These probiotic bacteria, found in live bio yogurt, produce butyrate, a short-chain fatty acid that provides energy for bowel-lining cells (colonocytes). Abnormal metabolism of butyrate has been suggested as a possible cause of ulcerative colitis, and probiotic bacteria help to maintain butyrate levels, so increasing your intake of live bio yogurt (or probiotic drinks) could help.

Butyrate levels are reduced by the action of sulphur compounds in the bowel – one reason why sulphur-rich foods may worsen ulcerative colitis symptoms.

## Foods to avoid

No foods consistently provoke symptoms in all sufferers (although it's a good idea to steer clear of the potential culprit foods listed in the

## USEFUL SUPPLEMENTS

- **A multivitamin and mineral** will guard against nutritional deficiencies – people with ulcerative colitis often have low levels of riboflavin ($B_2$), folate, beta-carotene, vitamin $B_{12}$, calcium, phosphorus, magnesium, selenium, zinc and vitamin D
- **Resistant fibre** found in oat bran and psyllium seed helps to boost bowel levels of beneficial probiotic bacteria
- **Omega-3 fish oils** (equivalent to EPA 3.2 g and DHA 2.4 g daily) have been shown to significantly improve symptoms
- **Aloe vera gel** contains a polysaccharide, acemannan, which boosts healing (avoid if pregnant or breastfeeding)
- **Frankincense** contains boswellic acids that reduce inflammation; studies from India, where it is an Ayurvedic treatment for ulcerative colitis, suggest it produces remission rates of 70–82 per cent
- **Fenugreek** is an aromatic herb also used in Ayurvedic medicine to treat ulcerative colitis
- **N-acetyl glucosamine** (1 g three times daily) has been shown to produce significant improvements in some cases of inflammatory bowel disease (avoid glucosamine sulphate, which is a source of sulphur)
- **Wheat grass** may be beneficial for ulcerative colitis, according to results from trials involving ingestion of wheat grass juice over a four-week period
- **Devil's claw extracts** are traditionally used to treat ulcerative colitis

Omega-3 fish oils can significantly improve symptoms.

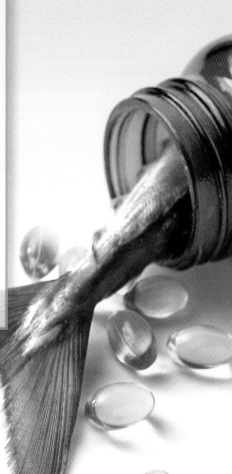

table on page 137, where possible). It's therefore important to identify and avoid the foods that provoke your own attacks. Some people find that they are sensitive to dairy and wheat produce, or that following a gluten-free diet is beneficial. Others are more likely to relapse following a high intake of red and processed meat, protein and alcohol.

Foods containing sulphites (added as a preservative) or caffeine appear to be particularly important triggers. Some sulphur compounds (such as hydrogen sulphide) have also been shown to damage the bowel lining and produce changes similar to those seen in ulcerative colitis. Although the bowel is usually able to detoxify these sulphur substances, this ability may be reduced in ulcerative colitis, as higher than normal bowel levels of sulphur compounds are detectable.

Avoid food additives numbered from E220 to E229, which are reserved for sulphites:

- E220 sulphur dioxide
- E221 sodium sulphite
- E222 sodium bisulphite (sodium hydrogen sulphite)
- E223 sodium metabisulphite
- E224 potassium metabisulphite
- E225 potassium sulphite
- E226 calcium sulphite
- E227 calcium hydrogen sulphite
- E228 potassium hydrogen sulphite

NOTE: 'Sulphur/sulphites' may also be spelled as 'sulfur/sulfites' on labels.

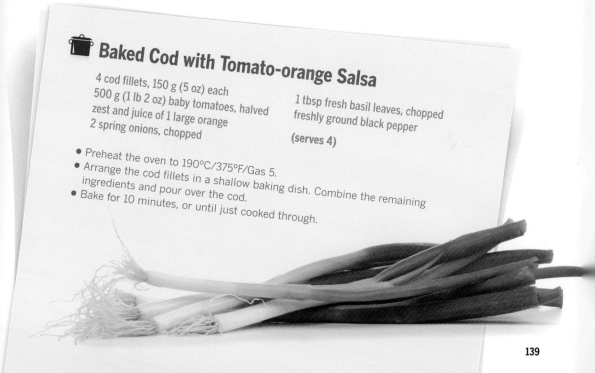

## 🍲 Baked Cod with Tomato-orange Salsa

4 cod fillets, 150 g (5 oz) each
500 g (1 lb 2 oz) baby tomatoes, halved
zest and juice of 1 large orange
2 spring onions, chopped

1 tbsp fresh basil leaves, chopped
freshly ground black pepper

(serves 4)

- Preheat the oven to 190°C/375°F/Gas 5.
- Arrange the cod fillets in a shallow baking dish. Combine the remaining ingredients and pour over the cod.
- Bake for 10 minutes, or until just cooked through.

# Crohn's disease

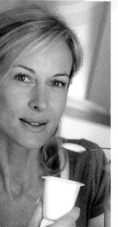

**Crohn's disease is a long-term** inflammatory condition of the bowel. Symptoms commonly appear between the ages of fifteen and thirty, or after the age of sixty, but can come on at any time. Following a specially devised diet appears to help manage symptoms.

Crohn's disease is associated with thickening, fissuring and ulceration of parts of the bowel wall. The site most usually affected is the end of the small intestine (terminal ileum), but it can affect any part of the gut from the mouth to the anus. Symptoms vary from mild to severe and include abdominal pain, fever, diarrhoea (which may contain blood), loss of appetite, lethargy, feeling unwell and loss of weight. Anaemia may result from poor nutrient absorption and long-term loss of blood from the inflamed bowel. Other parts of the body may also become inflamed, including the eyes, some joints, the spine (ankylosing spondylitis) and the skin, producing an eczema-like rash.

Symptoms tend to come and go over many years, but may slowly improve. Crohn's involves abnormal immune reactions, possibly to components in the diet or to an as yet unidentified bacterial, viral or parasitic infection. It is not contagious.

## Foods that can help

The LOFFLEX (low-fibre, fat-limited exclusion) diet designed for Crohn's disease includes the foods identified by bowel specialists as least likely to worsen symptoms (*see* table). It limits fat intake to around 50 g (2 oz) per day, and fibre to 10 g (⅓ oz), and excludes foods associated with relapses. One study found that over half of people who followed the

## Crohn's checklist

- **Keep a food and symptom diary** to help identify foods that you need to avoid long-term.
- **Don't rush your meals** – take time to chew well.
- **Drink plenty of fluids.**
- **Don't smoke:** smoking has an adverse effect on Crohn's disease, prompting more frequent and severe attacks.
- **Practise relaxation techniques** such as meditation and yoga, as stress can trigger flare-ups.
- **Try acupuncture:** traditional Chinese acupuncture has shown benefits in treating mild to moderately severe Crohn's disease.

# What causes it? CROHN'S DISEASE IS LINKED WITH:

• family history • unidentified infection • abnormal immune reactions • stress • smoking

| FOODS THAT ARE NOT ALLOWED | FOODS THAT ARE ALLOWED |
|---|---|
| Pork | Other lean meat and poultry |
| Fish in batter/oil/tomato | All other fish and shellfish |
| Milk (cow's, goat, sheep) and dairy products | Soy products |
| Wheat, rye, barley, millet, buckwheat, corn, oats | Rice, rice cakes, rice milk and rice cereals |
| Yeast | Tapioca, sago |
| Pulses, onion, tomatoes, sweetcorn | All other vegetables, including potatoes (no skins) |
| Citrus fruit, apples, bananas, dried fruits | All other fruits (no skins) |
| Vegetable, corn and nut oils | Sugar, honey, jam |
| Nuts and seeds | Fruit and herbal teas |
| Tea, coffee, alcohol, squashes, cola | Water |

## Rice cakes can be enjoyed as part of the LOFFLEX diet.

LOFFLEX diet were still free from symptoms after two years.

After following the LOFFLEX approach for two weeks, new 'test' foods are introduced, one at a time, every four days, as long as you remain symptom-free. Wheat products must be tested for seven days, as the onset of symptoms is often delayed after reintroducing this cereal.

If a test food causes side effects, continue to avoid it and wait until all symptoms have improved before testing another food. If no reactions occur, you then start testing a new food after four days. New foods are introduced in the following order: pork, oats, tea,

## Caution

The LOFFLEX diet should only be followed under the supervision of a medical nutritionist or dietician, and the full restriction part of the diet should not be followed for more than four weeks.

## USEFUL SUPPLEMENTS

- **A multivitamin and mineral supplement**, as Crohn's is associated with malnutrition
- **Probiotic supplements** are often helpful, as they promote a healthy balance of intestinal bacteria (some Bifidophilus probiotic strains – Bifidobacterium and Acidophilus – have been shown to prevent relapses of Crohn's symptoms, and to help maintain remission)
- **Omega-3 fish oils** can reduce bowel inflammation and prevent Crohn's flare-ups, according to some studies
- **Glucosamine supplements** have been shown to provide relief in some people after six weeks
- **Frankincense**, a resin containing boswellic acids, has an anti-inflammatory action; one eight-week trial found that Boswellia serrata extracts and the drug mesalazine reduced the Crohn's Disease Activity Index by similar amounts
- **Bromelain**, an extract from the pineapple plant, has been shown to decrease the production of inflammatory cytokines in colon cells obtained from people with Crohn's disease
- **Curcumin**, an antioxidant extract from turmeric spice, has an anti-inflammatory action, and has been reported to benefit patients with Crohn's disease
- **Devil's claw extracts** contain analgesic substances and are traditionally used to treat inflammatory bowel disease
- **Aloe vera juice** soothes and cleanses the bowel; select products declared aloin-free to avoid a laxative effect (avoid if pregnant or breastfeeding)

rye, eggs, onions, coffee, yeast, banana, apple, milk, butter/margarine, white wine, peas, chocolate, tomato, cheese, corn, citrus fruit, wheat, bread, yogurt, nuts and sweetcorn.

This diet can be nutritionally balanced if you eat a variety of allowed foods and you start introducing new 'test' foods within two to four weeks. If you find you need to avoid lots of foods because they worsen your symptoms, seek ongoing dietary advice (as always, it's best to make any significant dietary changes under the supervision of a medical nutritionist, to guard against nutrient deficiencies).

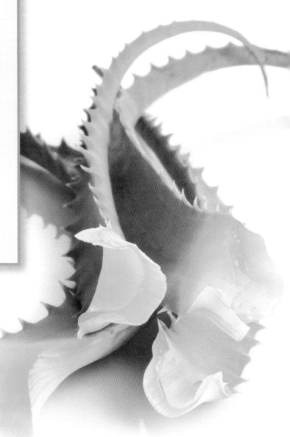

Aloe vera juice soothes and cleanses the bowel.

# Foods to avoid

Avoid any foods that seem to provoke your attacks (no single food consistently provokes symptoms in all people), plus those foods listed in the LOFFLEX table.

As with food allergies (*see* page 124) and irritable bowel syndrome (*see* page 132), food intolerance tests that identify raised levels of IgG antibodies against particular foods may help to identify foods you have an intolerance for, without having to follow a time-consuming elimination diet. Talk to a registered nutritionist to find out more.

## DID YOU KNOW?

**If avoiding** dairy products, you can (and should) obtain calcium from calcium-enriched soy milk and from green vegetables such as kale, spinach and broccoli.

 ## Lobster, Mango & Avocado Salad

bag of baby spinach leaves, washed
meat from one lobster, chopped
flesh of 1 ripe mango, chopped
flesh of 1 ripe avocado, chopped

1 tbsp fresh mint leaves, chopped
1 tsp powdered turmeric

(serves 4)

• Arrange the spinach leaves on four plates. Combine the remaining ingredients in a bowl, and then pile onto the leaves to serve.

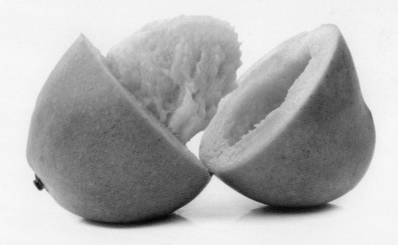

# Chronic fatigue syndrome (CFS)

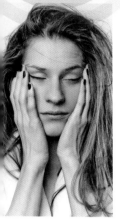

**CFS affects an estimated** one in 250 people and most commonly comes on between the mid-teens and mid-forties. Women are three times more likely to be affected than men. Beneficial dietary regimes vary from one person to another, so it's important to find what's right for you.

Also known as post-viral fatigue, chronic fatigue immune dysfunction syndrome and myalgic encephalopathy (muscle pain associated with neurological problems), CFS produces persistent physical and mental fatigue, muscle pain and twitching, and poor memory and concentration that is not relieved by sleep or rest. Those affected often feel unwell, with flu-like symptoms, sore throat and enlarged glands. Symptoms are disabling and typically worsen on exertion, following a characteristic delay that can vary from a few hours to a day or more. Unsurprisingly, many people also develop depression.

Most people with CFS experience fluctuating relapses interspersed with periods of normality. Some people make a full recovery, although this may take considerable time, while a few remain severely affected.

## Foods that can help

- **Follow a healthy, wholefood diet** that is as organic as possible, to avoid agricultural chemicals, colourings, preservatives and other food additives.
- **Maintain a healthy weight,** as difficulty with exercise may promote weight gain, and those whose appetite disappears or who feel too ill to eat properly may lose weight.
- **Eat little and often:** six small meals per day are better than three larger ones, as digestion and absorption appear to be impaired in people with CFS.
- **Increase intake of B vitamins,** as vitamin B status is often low; food sources include wholegrains, oats, beans, green leafy vegetables, oily fish, meat (especially pork and

## CFS checklist

- **Remain positive** about the chance of recovery.
- **Try cognitive behaviour therapy (CBT), graded exercise, gentle yoga or meditation,** as these may help.
- **Avoid smoking and alcohol.**

duck), nuts (especially walnuts), pomegranate, bio yogurt and fortified cereals.

In addition, some people with CFS have found benefit from following an anti-Candida dietary regime that provides very little sugar (*see* page 94), while others find that a low-animal-fat, high-fibre vegetarian diet is helpful.

## Foods to avoid

- **Avoid excessive caffeine,** as this worsens symptoms in some people.
- **Follow an elimination/challenge diet,** if you recognize that you have certain food or chemical intolerances, as this may help to pinpoint these (*see* food allergy & intolerance, pages 124–7).

### USEFUL SUPPLEMENTS

- **Co-enzyme Q10** is essential for oxygen uptake and production of energy in cells, and supplements may improve fatigue
- **Evening primrose and omega-3 fish oils** are rich in essential fatty acids and have been found to benefit up to 80 per cent of people with CFS, when taken in high doses
- **Magnesium** has been shown to improve tiredness and lack of energy
- **A vitamin B complex supplement** may help to guard against deficiency
- **Immune-stimulating herbs** such as echinacea, astragalus, lapacho or olive leaf extracts also have anti-viral actions and may be helpful (**note:** *these herbs are best taken under the supervision of a medical herbalist*)

## Beetroot, Pomegranate & Walnut Salad with Yogurt Dressing

1 large bag mixed salad leaves
2 cooked beetroot, peeled and chopped
handful of chopped walnuts
half a cucumber, chopped
2 spring onions, chopped
seeds from 1 pomegranate (optional)

For the dressing:
100 ml (3½ fl oz) low fat bio yogurt
2 tbsp wholegrain mustard
zest and juice of 1 unwaxed lemon
freshly ground black pepper

(serves 4)

- Scatter the salad leaves on a platter and arrange the beetroot, walnuts, cucumber, spring onions and pomegranate seeds (if using) on top.
- Mix the dressing ingredients well and drizzle over the salad.

145

# Lack of energy

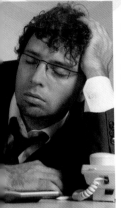

**Occasional lack of energy is normal**, but listlessness can creep up on you so you feel washed out and exhausted for much of the time. Adjusting your diet – together with other lifestyle changes – can help you to re-energize your life.

Lack of energy can result from an unidentified illness, but more often it is linked with stress and juggling different aspects of your life, such as working, looking after the home and taking care of other people, so that you find it difficult to put your feet up and look after your own health. Surveys suggest that one in three women and one in five men admit to feeling tired or lacking in energy on a regular basis, with one in ten adults admitting to feeling exhausted for a month or more.

## Associated medical conditions

If you feel lacking in energy for longer than two weeks, despite increasing your exercise levels, eating a healthy diet and improving your quality of sleep, see your doctor. Many illnesses start off this way. While only one in ten people are likely to have a medical cause for their symptoms, certain conditions need to be ruled out, such as anaemia, hormone imbalances (for example, underactive thyroid, diabetes), depression, side effects of medication, heart problems (such as irregular heartbeat, heart failure), hidden infection (for instance, of the heart valves), autoimmune disorders (for example, SLE), post-viral fatigue and cancer (the latter affecting less than one in 100 people with lack of energy and no other symptoms).

Carbon-monoxide poisoning could also be a cause, especially if symptoms are accompanied by headache and rapidly clear on breathing fresh air. (If you think this may be the case, get your household appliances checked by a professional, and make sure there is adequate ventilation in your home.)

## Energy-boosting checklist

- **Exercise daily in the fresh air** to boost your metabolism.
- **Find time for rest and relaxation** – sit quietly reading or meditating, or listen to music.
- **Lose any excess weight.**
- **Avoid working long hours** without a break.
- **Get back in control of your life** – say 'no' to unreasonable demands.
- **Go to bed early,** and keep a window slightly open to allow oxygen to circulate.
- **Take a power nap** when you can during the day.

## What causes it? LACK OF ENERGY IS LINKED WITH:

• stress • anxiety • over-exertion • poor diet • inactivity • hormone changes • working long hours • poor-quality sleep • some illnesses

## Foods that can help

• **Kick-start the day with porridge:** researchers in Australia have found that athletes following an oat-based diet for three weeks enjoyed a 4 per cent increase in stamina.

• **Follow a low- to moderate-GI diet,** based on high-fibre foods such as fresh fruit, vegetables, beans, nuts, seeds, root vegetables and wholegrains (wholemeal bread, wholewheat pasta, pearl barley, quinoa, teff, brown rice).

• **Eat regular meals spaced evenly throughout the day,** to ensure blood glucose levels remain relatively stable.

• **Increase intake of B vitamins,** needed for energy production in cells; food sources include lean meat, eggs, oats, yeast extracts, dairy and brown rice.

• **Choose healthy snacks** such as oatcakes, rice cakes, nut butters,

Kick-start the day with porridge.

### LOOK AFTER NUMBER ONE

There are times when you need to put yourself first – and if you're lacking in energy or tired all the time, this is one of them! Don't neglect your own needs.

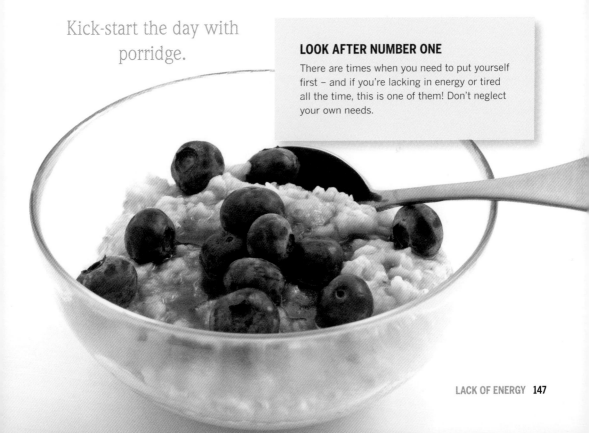

hummus, guacamole, vegetable sticks, fruit and low-fat yogurt.

- **Select iron-rich foods,** if anaemia is a possibility (for example, linked to heavy periods, recent pregnancy, poor diet), such as red meat, fish (especially sardines), wheatgerm, bread made with fortified flour, eggs, dark green leafy vegetables (such as kale, spinach, parsley), prunes and other dried fruit. Increasing your intake of vitamin C will boost iron absorption, so drink a glass of fresh orange juice with a boiled egg for breakfast, instead of having a mug of tea (iron absorption is blocked by tannins).
- **Drink plenty of fluids** to keep hydrated – even mild dehydration can cause fatigue.

# Foods to avoid

- **Avoid stodgy, fatty foods** such as chips, pastries, cakes, sweet biscuits, doughnuts, pies and fry-ups. Eating a fatty breakfast is associated with more fatigue, a lower mood and less alertness during the morning than eating a low-fat, high-fibre, carbohydrate-based breakfast. And, if you then follow a fatty breakfast with a fatty lunch, you'll feel lacking in energy all day.
- **Don't over-eat:** this drains blood away from your brain to the digestive system, which makes you feel tired.
- **Avoid foods containing simple sugars,** such as cakes, chocolate, white bread and pasta, as, while these may provide a rapid energy high, your body responds by

Choose healthy snacks instead of stodgy, fatty foods.

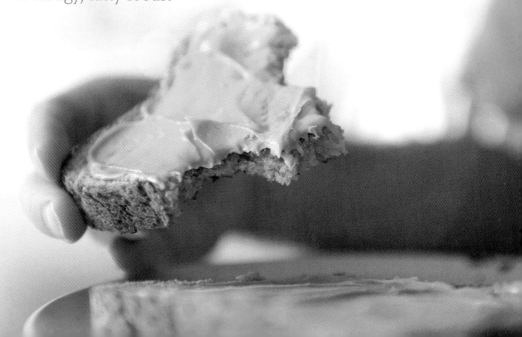

secreting insulin to bring blood glucose levels down. This can cause an energy crash a few hours after eating (making you likely to nod off after a lunch of white-bread sandwiches and a sugary soft drink).

- **Cut back on caffeine.** Caffeine is now recognized as one of the great energy-drainers: in the short term it gives a quick, alerting boost, but in the long term it can lead to restlessness, insomnia, headache, anxiety and fatigue. Make sure you cut back slowly, to avoid caffeine withdrawal symptoms.
- **Avoid excess alcohol,** as this makes you feel tired. Try avoiding alcohol for a few weeks to see if symptoms improve (if you find this difficult, seek medical advice).

## USEFUL SUPPLEMENTS

- **A multivitamin and mineral** will guard against nutrient deficiencies
- **B group vitamins**, alpha-lipoic acid and l-carnitine are needed for energy production in cells
- **Magnesium** is essential for energy production but is often lacking in the diet
- **Co-enzyme Q10** improves physical energy levels and endurance
- **Ginkgo biloba** boosts blood flow to the brain, improving mental energy, memory and alertness
- **Guarana** contains tetramethyl xanthene similar to caffeine (a trimethyl xanthene), and can relieve fatigue with less of the side effects associated with caffeine
- **Korean ginseng** boosts physical energy, prevents fatigue and improves endurance
- **Siberian ginseng** improves physical and mental energy levels, especially under stress

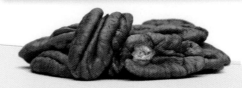

 **Pecan Nut Roast**

2 tbsp olive, rapeseed or hempseed oil
1 large onion, chopped
2 cloves garlic, chopped
handful fresh herbs (parsley, thyme, marjoram, sage), chopped
200 g (7 oz) wholemeal breadcrumbs

150 g (5 oz) pecan nuts, finely chopped
1 large egg, beaten
150 ml (¼ pt) vegetable stock or water
zest and juice of 1 lemon
freshly ground black pepper

**(serves 4)**

- Preheat the oven to 200°C/400°F/Gas 6. Line a 450 g (1 lb) loaf tin with non-stick baking paper.
- Sauté the onion and garlic in the oil until soft. Combine with all the remaining ingredients and mix well. Pile into the lined loaf tin.
- Bake for 30 minutes until lightly brown. Allow to cool slightly in the tin, then turn out.

# Anaemia

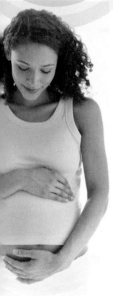

**Anaemia affects an estimated** 23 per cent of the population across Europe, though is significantly less common in the US, where fewer than one in fifty people are affected. The most common causes of anaemia are due to lack of iron, folic acid or vitamin $B_{12}$ in the diet, so dietary changes are essential in order to combat this condition.

Anaemia literally means 'without blood' and relates to having low levels of the red pigment haemoglobin within your circulating red blood cells. Haemoglobin is vital for carrying oxygen around the body, and when levels fall your cells do not receive enough oxygen for their needs. Symptoms include paleness, tiredness, lack of energy, dizziness, recurrent infections (especially Candida), sore tongue and mouth, shortness of breath and even angina. Pernicious anaemia occurs when the stomach stops producing a substance called intrinsic factor, which is needed for the absorption of vitamin $B_{12}$ in the small intestine.

Iron-deficiency anaemia is common among certain vulnerable groups, including breast-fed infants, toddlers, adolescents, menstruating and pregnant women, and the elderly.

## Foods that can help

Dietary sources of iron include shellfish, red meats, sardines, wheatgerm, wholemeal bread, egg yolk, green vegetables, nuts, wholegrains, dried fruit and fortified breakfast cereals. The form of iron found in red meat (haem iron) is up to ten times more easily absorbed than the non-haem iron in vegetables; meat eaters are therefore less prone to iron-deficiency anaemia than non-meat eaters. Plant-based iron is absorbed more easily if eaten together with a source of vitamin C such as fresh orange juice.

---

### USEFUL SUPPLEMENTS

- **Iron supplements** in the form of amino acid chelates (such as ferrous bisglycinate) are better absorbed and better tolerated than inorganic ferrous sulphate
- **Vitamin $B_{12}$** is also available as an oral spray or sublingual lozenges for absorption in the mouth (to bypass any lack of intrinsic factor in the gut)

**Note:** *Excess iron is toxic, so keep any supplements out of the sight and reach of children.*

---

- poor nutrition • heavy periods • hidden blood loss (such as a bleeding peptic ulcer)
- recycling blood cells too quickly (for example, sickle cell disease) • kidney disease
- bone marrow disease • malabsorption of dietary nutrients

Folate is found mainly in green leafy vegetables and in fortified cereals, while food sources of vitamin $B_{12}$ include liver, kidney, oily fish (especially sardines), white fish, red meats, eggs and dairy products. No plants contain consistent amounts of $B_{12}$, although vegetarian supplements derived from blue-green algae or cultured micro-organisms are available.

 **Beef, Spinach & Tomato Stew**

400 g (14 oz) lean stewing beef, cubed
1 large onion, sliced
handful of fresh herbs (such as thyme, parsley, marjoram), chopped
1 clove garlic, crushed
300 ml (½ pt) stock made with low-salt bouillon cube

1 x 400 g (14 oz) can chopped tomatoes
1 tbsp tomato purée
freshly ground black pepper
1 bag fresh baby spinach leaves, washed and drained

(serves 4)

- Preheat the oven to 180°C/350°F/Gas 4.
- Place the beef, onion, herbs, garlic and stock into a hob-proof casserole dish. Bring to the boil, then cover and put in the oven for 30 minutes.
- Add the chopped tomatoes and the purée, stir well and cook for another hour.
- Season with black pepper, and add the spinach leaves so they wilt into the stew. Serve with brown rice and salad.

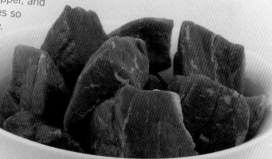

Meat eaters are less prone to iron-deficiency anaemia than non-meat eaters.

# Thyroid problems

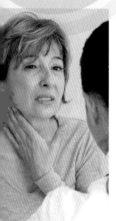

**As many as one in twelve** women are affected by hypothyroidism (underactive thyroid), while 2–5 per cent of women are affected by hyperthyroidism (overactive thyroid). Both conditions are ten times less common in males. Different foods can help, depending on which condition you have.

The thyroid is a butterfly-shaped gland in the base of the neck, just in front of the trachea (windpipe). It produces two iodine-containing hormones – thyroxine (T4) and triiodothyronine (T3) – that boost metabolism by increasing the speed at which cells work.

In hypothyroidism, too few of these hormones are produced; conversely, in hyperthyroidism (also known as thyrotoxicosis), too many are produced. Many hypothyroidism cases are sub-clinical (not obvious); an obviously underactive thyroid affects around one in fifty women.

## Hypothyroidism

Most cases of hypothyroidism are due to an autoimmune condition in which the immune system makes antibodies aimed against thyroid proteins, leading to chronic autoimmune thyroiditis. Although many people have no obvious symptoms, the condition can cause swelling of the thyroid gland to produce a goitre, with a sensation of fullness in the neck, trouble swallowing and, occasionally, discomfort or pain in the neck or chest. Initially, these antibodies may cause inflammation and transient symptoms of an overactive thyroid gland, but more usually the condition slowly progresses to cause symptoms linked with low levels of thyroid hormone (hypothyroidism). Other cases result from treatment of an overactive thyroid gland or, in some parts of the world, from severe dietary deficiency of iodine, selenium or zinc.

## Thyroid checklist

- Take tablets at least two hours apart, if you are taking both thyroxine hormone tablets and iron supplements, as the absorption of thyroxine is reduced by iron.
- Talk to your doctor about also taking T3 hormone replacement, if you still have symptoms of hypothyroidism despite taking thyroxine (T4) (although this is controversial in the UK, it is common in the US).

## What causes it? THYROID PROBLEMS ARE LINKED WITH:
- family history • coeliac disease and other autoimmune conditions including diabetes
- certain drugs • lack of iodine (hypothyroidism) • excess iodine (hyperthyroidism)

### DID YOU KNOW**?**

**In people** who have both coeliac and thyroid disease, following a gluten-free diet improves both conditions.

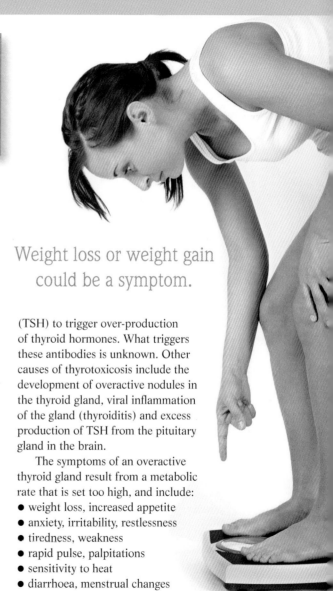

Smoking cigarettes has also been linked with an increased risk of developing hypothyroidism.

The symptoms of an underactive thyroid gland are due to a metabolism that is set too slow, and include:
- lack of energy, general slowing down
- muscle cramps and weakness
- increasing weight
- feeling the cold
- dry skin, brittle hair, loss of outer third of eyebrows
- thickening of tissues in the face and limbs
- slow pulse
- constipation, heavy periods
- a deepening voice which may seem slurred

## Hyperthyroidism

The most common cause of an overactive thyroid is Grave's disease, an autoimmune condition in which thyroid-stimulating antibodies bind to thyroid cell receptors and mimic the action of thyroid stimulating hormone

Weight loss or weight gain could be a symptom.

(TSH) to trigger over-production of thyroid hormones. What triggers these antibodies is unknown. Other causes of thyrotoxicosis include the development of overactive nodules in the thyroid gland, viral inflammation of the gland (thyroiditis) and excess production of TSH from the pituitary gland in the brain.

The symptoms of an overactive thyroid gland result from a metabolic rate that is set too high, and include:
- weight loss, increased appetite
- anxiety, irritability, restlessness
- tiredness, weakness
- rapid pulse, palpitations
- sensitivity to heat
- diarrhoea, menstrual changes

## Foods that can help

- **Follow a diet free from sugar and refined foods,** as this can improve thyroid function.
- **Eat more selenium-rich foods;** dietary sources include wheatgerm, Brazil nuts, fish, wholegrain cereals, mushrooms, onions and garlic. Selenium is needed to regulate the production of the most active thyroid hormone, T3; thyroid tissue therefore has the highest selenium content per gram of any organ in the body. In parts of the world where soil levels of selenium and iodine are low (including the UK), the risk of developing an underactive thyroid gland is especially high.

*If you have hypothyroidism:*
- **Eat sources of iodine,** such as fish, seafood, eggs, meat, milk and iodized salt. A study of vegetarians published in the *British Journal of Medicine* found that 63 per cent of females and 36 per cent of males had inadequate iodine intake.

*If you have hyperthyroidism:*
- **Eat more goitrogen-containing foods:** goitrogens block conversion of T4 hormone to T3 (the most active form), so can be beneficial if you have hyperthyroidism. Food sources include Brussels sprouts, broccoli, cabbage, cauliflower, kale, turnips, pak choy, Chinese leaves, collard greens, horseradish, radishes, swede (rutabaga), cassava and soybeans.

### HORMONE REPLACEMENT THERAPY

Hypothyroidism is treated with thyroid hormone replacement therapy to restore the level of thyroid stimulating hormone (TSH, made in the pituitary) to within the normal range. Some endocrinologists believe that complete well-being is only restored when your thyroxine level is towards the upper limit of normal, and your TSH level is slightly suppressed. This is something you need to discuss with your doctor, so that you minimize the risk of side effects (symptoms of an overactive thyroid) while optimizing your metabolic rate to reduce weight gain and lack of energy.

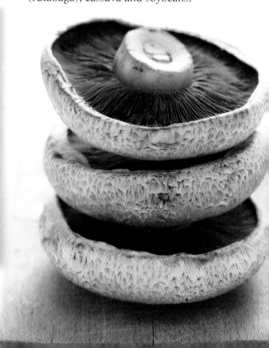

## Foods to avoid

*If you have hypothyroidism:*
- Avoid eating excessive amounts of goitrogen-containing foods (*see* list opposite, under foods that can help for hyperthyroidism).

*If you have hyperthyroidism:*
- Avoid iodized salt and stimulants such as coffee, tea and other caffeinated drinks, which speed up the metabolism.

### USEFUL SUPPLEMENTS

- **A multivitamin and mineral supplement** that includes iodine, selenium and zinc will support thyroid function (avoid iodine if hyperthyroid), as vitamins and minerals are used up more quickly by the increased metabolic rate
- **Kelp** is a naturally rich source of iodine, where an underactive thyroid is thought to be linked with low iodine intake (avoid if hyperthyroid)
- **Evening primrose oil** and **omega-3 fish oils** help to avoid essential-fatty-acid deficiencies
- **Valerian** and **rhodiola** are calming herbs that can help to reduce the anxiety and nervousness associated with hyperthyroidism

 ## Halibut with Mushrooms & Shallots

2 tbsp olive, rapeseed or hempseed oil
4 shallots, chopped
16 button mushrooms, halved
4 cloves garlic, crushed
4 halibut steaks
50 ml (2 fl oz) white wine

zest and juice of 1 unwaxed lemon
1 tsp cornflour
freshly ground black pepper
parsley to garnish

(serves 4)

- Heat the oil in a large, flat pan and sauté the shallots, mushrooms and garlic until softened.
- Place the halibut steaks on top, and pour over the white wine and lemon juice/zest. Cover and cook for 5 minutes, then turn the fillets over and cook for another 5 minutes, or until the flesh is set. Remove the fish and keep warm.
- Dissolve the cornflour in a little extra white wine or water. Stir into the mushroom and onion sauce and simmer until thickened to your desired consistency. Season with black pepper, pour over the halibut and serve garnished with parsley.

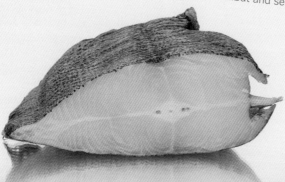

# Cancer

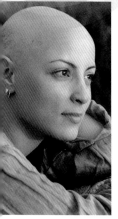

**Cancer is the leading cause** of death worldwide. Your lifetime risk of receiving a cancer diagnosis is one in three, and your chance of dying from cancer before the age of seventy-five is currently one in nine (higher if you smoke, or if cancer runs in your family). Eating more foods with anti-cancer properties increases your chances of keeping this prevalent disease at bay.

A cancer develops when a single cell divides repeatedly, rather than just occasionally to replace worn out cells. It produces abnormal copies of itself that do not respond to the usual instructions to stop growing. If the immune system doesn't recognize and destroy these abnormal cells, they continue to divide and invade surrounding tissues. Once the tumour reaches a certain size, abnormal cells may break away and spread through blood and lymph vessels to other parts of the body. These secondary tumours (metastases) most commonly take root and continue to grow in the lung, bone, liver and brain.

The number of cancer deaths worldwide doubled between 1975 and 2000, will double again by 2020, and is expected to triple by 2030.

## Symptom checklist

**Persistent symptoms that shouldn't be ignored include:**

- a change in bowel habit
- urinary difficulties
- recurrent heartburn
- a nagging cough or shortness of breath
- pain or discomfort that keeps coming back
- weight loss for no apparent reason
- unexpected blood loss from any orifice (including post-menopausal and post-coital bleeding)
- difficulty swallowing
- feeling full despite eating very little
- hoarse voice or sore throat lasting more than three weeks
- any persistent health problem that worries you

## Foods that can help

There are, of course, no guarantees, but you can help to give yourself a fighting chance by incorporating more of the following beneficial foods into your diet.

- **Follow a plant-based, antioxidant-rich diet,** as this offers numerous anti-cancer benefits. Fruit and

## What causes it? CANCER IS LINKED WITH:

- family history • ill-understood interactions between our genes, environment, diet and lifestyle
- smoking • alcohol • obesity • lack of exercise • air pollution • work-place carcinogens • indoor smoke from solid fuels • hepatitis viruses • some types of human wart (papilloma) virus

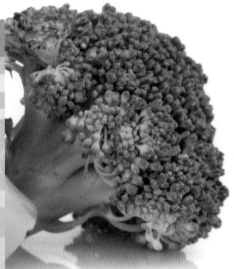

| FOOD | ANTI-CANCER COMPOUNDS |
|------|------------------------|
| Broccoli | sulphoraphane |
| Cabbage family | isothiocyanates |
| Tomatoes | lycopene |
| Garlic | allicin |
| Mushrooms | lentinan |
| Onions, leeks, apples | flavonoids |
| Peppers | capsaicins |
| Celery, parsley | apigenin |
| Cherries, berries, grapes | ellagic acid |
| Citrus fruits | limonene, hesperidin, limonoids |
| Brazil nuts | selenium |
| Soybeans, alfalfa | isoflavones |
| Oily fish | eicosapentaenoic acid |
| Seeds | lignans |
| Green/black tea | catechins |

vegetables provide phytochemicals – non-nutrient substances such as flavonoids, phenols and terpenes – which appear to protect against cancer. Eat at least 450 g (1 lb) of these per day (not counting potatoes), and select a wide variety, such as tomatoes, citrus fruits, berries, peppers, carrots, broccoli, cabbage and beans (*see also* table above).

- **Seek out selenium,** which is needed to make powerful anti-cancer enzymes in the body. In parts of the world where soil selenium levels are low, the incidence of cancer increases two- to six-fold. The best food sources are Brazil nuts, fish, poultry, meats (especially game), wholegrains, mushrooms, onions, garlic, broccoli and cabbage.

- **Increase intake of isoflavones** – weak plant hormones that damp down the effects of excess human oestrogens by blocking the same receptors. In Asia, where intakes of soy isoflavones are 50–100 mg per day, compared with typical Western intakes of just 2–5 mg per day, the risk of hormone-related cancers, such as those of the breast and prostate, is significantly lower.

DID YOU KNOW?

**At least** 40 per cent of cancers can be prevented by lifestyle changes. Smoking is the single greatest preventable cause.

Isoflavones are found in beans, lentils, chickpeas, fennel, nuts and seeds.

- **Consume more calcium and vitamin D** – these may protect against colon cancer. Good sources of calcium include milk, cheese, yogurt and dark green leafy vegetables such as kale and spinach. Sources of vitamin D include oily fish, fish liver oils, animal liver, fortified margarine, eggs, butter and fortified milk and cereals.

- **Reach for the garlic:** people who eat the most garlic appear least likely to develop stomach, bowel and prostate cancers.
- **Drink more tea:** green tea polyphenols have been found to help protect against cancers of the bladder, oesophagus, pancreas, ovaries, and possibly cervix.
- **Eat more fibre.** There is conflicting evidence regarding fibre and bowel cancer but, in general, a good fibre intake helps to move waste through the digestive tract, so potential toxins have less time to affect intestinal cells. Good sources include wholegrain cereals and breads, prunes, berries, kidney beans and other legumes, fresh fruits and vegetables and brown rice.
- **Maintain a healthy weight** for your height and exercise daily.

## Foods to avoid

A diet high in fat, calories, processed carbohydrates, salt, alcohol and smoked or chargrilled foods, and low in antioxidants and fibre, will increase the risk of cancer. Excess dietary fat is considered a leading contributor to bowel cancer, as it triggers the release of bile acids into the intestines. When these reach the colon, the excess acids are converted to secondary substances that promote tumour growth.

- **Cut back on fat overall,** and focus on obtaining 'good' fats such as monounsaturates (olive, rapeseed, avocado and nut oils) plus omega-3s (such as fish and flaxseed oils).

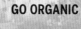

**GO ORGANIC**

**Agricultural residues** are found in non-organically grown produce, and 90 per cent of fungicides, 60 per cent of herbicides and 30 per cent of insecticides have potential cancer-causing properties.

- **Eat less red meat,** and less cured and processed meats such as sausages, bacon, burgers and ham – especially if fried, chargrilled or barbecued (burning meat produces chemicals that are linked with bowel cancer).
- **Limit intake of salt-cured, salt-pickled and smoked foods.**
- **Cut back on refined-carbohydrate foods** such as cakes and biscuits.
- **Avoid excess alcohol** – drink in moderation.

## USEFUL SUPPLEMENTS

No supplements should be taken specifically to protect against cancer. However, if you are taking them for other reasons, a number of vitamins, minerals and foodstuffs have shown anti-cancer properties in some studies, though the evidence is not definitive. These include selenium, soy isoflavones, vitamins C and D, folic acid, green tea, garlic, tomato extracts and some Asian mushrooms (such as reishi, shiitake, maitake, coriolus).

**Caution:** *If you have cancer, always seek medical advice before taking supplements.*

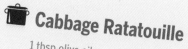 **Cabbage Ratatouille**

1 tbsp olive oil
1 red onion, chopped
1 leek, chopped and washed
4 cloves garlic, crushed
1 stick celery, chopped
1 red pepper, deseeded and sliced
half a cabbage, shredded
1 aubergine, chopped
1 courgette, chopped
handful of button mushrooms, halved

zest and juice of 1 unwaxed lemon
4 beef tomatoes, chopped
1 tbsp tomato purée
150 ml (¼ pt) red wine or vegetable stock
handful of mixed fresh herbs (such as parsley, basil, thyme, rosemary, coriander), chopped
freshly ground black pepper

**(serves 4)**

- Heat the olive oil in a large pan and sauté the onion, leek, garlic and celery until soft. Add the red pepper, cabbage and aubergine and stir fry for 5 minutes.
- Add all the remaining ingredients, cover and simmer gently, with the lid on, for 30 minutes. Stir occasionally, adding water if more liquid is needed. Season with black pepper, and serve.

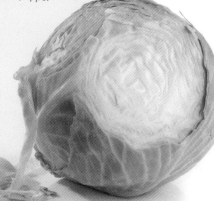

# Colds & flu

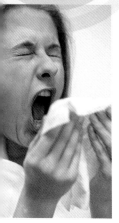

**Cold and flu viruses spread** from person to person through coughing, sneezing, talking and even when shaking hands. But if you follow a healthy diet and lifestyle, you are far less likely to succumb.

Over a hundred different viruses cause symptoms of the common cold, making it the most common disease in humans. Adults get an average of two to three colds per year, while children sometimes suffer as many as ten, partly because of increased exposure in nurseries and schools, and partly because their immunity is not yet primed against them. Flu symptoms initially resemble a cold but quickly get significantly worse.

## Foods that can help

The immune system is most active in the lining of the gut, so make sure you're giving your gut what it needs to stay healthy.

- **Eat a healthy, wholefood diet** providing at least five servings of fresh fruit and vegetables daily (preferably more).
- **Increase intake of omega-3s,** found in oily fish, nuts and seeds – these reduce susceptibility to allergies and inflammation.
- **Have an apple a day:** these contain soluble fibre and antioxidant flavonoids that activate immune cells and reduce inflammation.
- **Enjoy more elderberries,** which supply natural antiviral substances shown to reduce the severity and duration of cold and flu infections.
- **Cook with onions and garlic,** as these have antiviral properties.

| SYMPTOM | COMMON COLD | FLU |
| --- | --- | --- |
| Headache | uncommon | pronounced |
| Blocked nose | usual | sometimes |
| Sneezing | usual | sometimes |
| Sore throat | common | sometimes |
| Cough | mild to moderate | mild to severe |
| General aches and pains | slight | severe |
| Extreme exhaustion | never | pronounced |
| Weakness | mild | severe; can last 2–3 weeks |
| Fever | slight or none | usually 39°C (102.2°F) or higher for 3–4 days |

## What causes it? COLDS & FLU ARE LINKED WITH:

- rhinoviruses (which are more active in colder months) • echo and Coxsackie viruses (which are more active in summer) • influenza type A and B viruses • air-conditioning (which can dry your nasal lining to help viruses enter your nose more easily) • poor hygiene

- **Step up the selenium,** needed to make antibodies and to stimulate natural killer cells that fight infections. Flu symptoms are more severe in people with selenium deficiency. The richest dietary source is Brazil nuts – eat a couple a day.
- **Ensure good levels of vitamin D** from fish liver oils, animal liver, fortified margarine, eggs, butter, fortified milk and supplements.
- **Get enough zinc:** optimum zinc levels help to shorten the duration of a cold. Dietary sources include most meats, shellfish, nuts and seeds (especially pumpkin seeds) and fortified cereals.
- **Have a daily probiotic drink or supplement** to prime immunity.

If symptoms develop, drink plenty of warm fluids and eat simple, soothing foods such as soup, yogurt or scrambled eggs on bread.

### Cold and flu checklist

- **Avoid stress** and get enough sleep.
- **Exercise regularly** but avoid over-training.
- **Avoid cigarette smoke** and other air pollutants, where possible.
- **Avoid people with obvious cold symptoms** and don't shake their hand!
- **Wash hands regularly** and use antibacterial hand wipes/sprays and antiviral tissues.
- **Wipe down door handles,** as viruses can survive for many hours.
- **Seek advice from your doctor or pharmacist** regarding flu vaccinations, available to help protect people at particular risk.

 ### Elderberry Purée

150 g (5 oz) ripe elderberries, washed and de-stemmed
250 g (9 oz) apples, peeled, cored and chopped

zest and juice of 1 lemon
100 ml (3½ oz) water
stevia to taste

(serves 4)

- Place all ingredients except the stevia in a pan and bring to the boil. Simmer for 10 minutes.
- Remove from the heat and whizz in a blender until smooth. Sweeten to taste with stevia (a natural sweetener with zero calories) or your chosen sweetener. Stir the purée into yogurt, porridge or muesli, serve as a coulis with any dessert, or with roast or cold meats. Alternatively, dilute with water and freeze to make ice lollies.

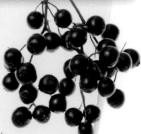

# Bad breath

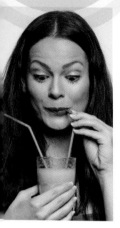

**Bad breath, or halitosis,** is a common problem that's difficult to spot yourself, and one even your best friend may be embarrassed to warn you about. Watching what you consume (and how you consume it) and keeping your mouth healthy helps to combat this condition.

The usual cause is a build-up of bacterial plaque in the mouth; these produce over 100 unpleasant-smelling gases and volatile chemicals. People with gum disease are four times more likely to have bad breath than others. If you have redness or swelling of the gums round your teeth, or if your gums bleed when brushing, you may have gingivitis (infected gums). If ignored, this will spread to involve the jawbone (periodontitis) and cause bad breath that's detectable from several feet away.

Saliva washes the mouth clean, and contains antibodies that reduce bacterial infection as well as enzymes that break down food trapped between the teeth. It also contains minerals that help to neutralize the acids produced by plaque bacteria. Lack of saliva increases the chance of bad breath and tooth decay, so if you suffer from a dry mouth, use an artificial saliva spray.

## Protect your enamel

Tooth enamel is the hardest substance in the body, but readily dissolves in dietary acids with a pH (measure of acidity) of less than 5.5. Once enamel dissolves away, the softer, underlying parts of the tooth start to decay, and this can cause bad breath. The table below gives examples of foods and drinks that harm your teeth on prolonged contact.

## Foods that can help

- **Decrease the frequency with which you consume acidic food or drink,** and consume them quickly, rather than chewing or sipping daintily. Don't avoid fruit and fruit juices altogether, as they form a vital part of a healthy diet. Using a straw

| FOOD/DRINK | PH |
|---|---|
| Black tea | 4.2 |
| Mayonnaise | 3.8–4.0 |
| Tomatoes | 3.7–4.7 |
| Grapes | 3.3–4.5 |
| Apples | 2.9–3.5 |
| Orange juice | 2.8–4.0 |
| Fizzy cola drinks | 2.7 |
| Vinegar | 2.4–3.4 |
| Black coffee | 2.4–3.3 |
| Lemon/Lime juice | 1.8–2.4 |

## What causes it? BAD BREATH IS LINKED WITH:

• bacterial plaque • dry mouth • nasal problems (previous fracture/surgery, post-nasal mucus drip) • sinusitis • long-term lung infection

positioned towards the back of your mouth lessens the contact time between fluids and your teeth, and may help reduce erosion caused by soft drinks.

• **Rehydrate your mouth regularly** by sipping water, and sluice your mouth out after drinking tea, coffee, cola, sports drinks and alcoholic drinks.

• **Eat more foods containing calcium,** such as cheese and other dairy products, as these protect against acid erosion, and select fruit juices fortified with added calcium; this decreases their erosive potential. Dental experts suggest holding a piece of cheese in your mouth for a few minutes after eating a fruit salad, to counter the acidic effects.

• **Eat peppermints or parsley, or chew sugar-free gum,** to help mask breath odours from eating onions and garlic.

• **Avoid high protein diets,** which contribute to mouth odour.

## Fresh-breath checklist

• **Invest in an electric toothbrush** that cleans with high-frequency sonic vibrations or which has a rotating head.

• **Use dental floss/tape regularly;** note where food becomes trapped between your teeth and tell your dentist.

• **Use a mouthwash** that binds bacteria and removes them in visible clumps, or which oxidizes sulphur molecules to eliminate bad breath.

• **Visit a dental hygienist at least twice a year** to have gum pockets cleaned and scale removed.

• **Consider Co-enzyme Q10 tablets and topical hyaluronic acid gel,** which can reverse gum inflammation and promote healing of gum disease.

*Chew sugar-free gum to help mask breath odours.*

## Cheesy Cottage Cheese

500 g (1 lb 2 oz) natural, low-fat cottage cheese
handful of grated cheddar cheese

handful of chives, snipped
freshly ground black pepper

(serves 4)

• Combine all ingredients and season to taste. Serve piled on baby spinach leaves as a salad, or in brown bread (another good source of calcium) as a sandwich filler.

# Migraine

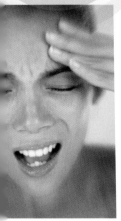

**Migraine is estimated to affect** as many as one in ten adults, with three times more women affected than men. Symptoms usually begin at puberty and cause recurrent attacks until middle age, when they often disappear. Eating magnesium-rich foods and identifying triggers can help.

Migraine is a severe headache, described as a throbbing, pulsating or hammering pain on one side of the head, often around one eye. Nausea and vomiting can also occur. Some people experience a warning 'aura' up to an hour before an attack, which may include visual symptoms (for example, shimmering or flashing lights, strange zig-zag shapes, blind spots), numbness or tingling on one side of the face, and sometimes speech difficulties. Migraine is associated with widening of blood vessels in the brain, so nerve tissue becomes congested.

## Foods that can help

- **Follow a well-balanced diet,** avoiding refined carbohydrates, fasting or skipping meals.
- **Consume more olive and fish oils** – these have been shown to reduce the frequency, duration and severity of migraine.
- **Eat magnesium-rich foods,** such as spinach, sweet potatoes and wholegrains, as magnesium levels are consistently low in people with migraine.
- **Reduce fat intake:** studies show that cutting dietary fat from 66 g to 28 g (2¼ oz to 1 oz) daily significantly reduces migraine frequency, intensity, duration and the need for medication.

### TRIGGER FOODS

Many foods are known to trigger migraine, especially milk and chocolate (the prime culprits, at 43 and 29 per cent), German sausages, cheese, fish, wine, coffee, garlic and eggs. Other reported dietary triggers include beans, beef, citrus fruits, corn, fried foods,

---

## USEFUL SUPPLEMENTS

- **Turmeric** is a traditional Ayurvedic treatment for migraine: add 1 tsp powdered turmeric to warm water, or take turmeric extracts (curcumin) in capsule form
- **Magnesium supplements** can reduce the frequency of attacks
- **Vitamin B₂ (riboflavin)** taken in high dose (400 mg) has been found to halve the frequency of attacks

## What causes it? MIGRAINE IS LINKED WITH:

● family history ● tiredness ● fatigue ● changes in stress levels ● dehydration ● certain foods ● caffeine ● menstruation ● extreme emotions such as anger or excitement

nuts, pork, shellfish, tea, tomatoes, caffeine and artificial sweeteners.

Follow an elimination diet that avoids common dietary triggers for two weeks, then re-introduce excluded foods, one at a time, to see if any trigger your migraine. Keep a food diary to pinpoint associations for at least two weeks, or long enough to cover three migraine attacks (bear in mind that trigger foods are usually eaten/drunk 24–48 hours before the migraine occurs). All foods related to suspects must be eliminated (for instance, all dairy products if milk is suspected), and other factors such as work stress and stage of menstrual cycle must also be taken into account.

## Migraine checklist

● **Drink sufficient fluids** to keep hydrated.
● **Eat little and often** to reduce hypoglycemia.
● **Try to identify your triggers** and, where possible, avoid them.

Keep a food diary ···

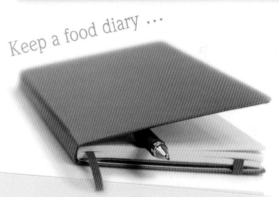

##  Sweet Potato & Spinach Stir-fry

2 tbsp olive oil
2 large, sweet potatoes, peeled and cubed
1 tsp turmeric powder (fresh)
100 ml (3½ fl oz) water

1 red onion, chopped
1 bag baby spinach leaves, washed
freshly ground black pepper

(serves 4)

● Fry the sweet potato cubes in olive oil for 10 minutes.
● Add the turmeric, water and red onion, and cook over a gentle heat, stirring, until the water has evaporated and the potatoes are tender.
● Add the baby spinach leaves and heat until they wilt. Season with black pepper and serve.

# Prostate enlargement

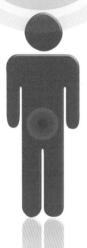

**By the age of sixty**, half of all men are affected by an enlarged prostate (though not all experience troublesome symptoms). Dietary factors have been found to play a key role in prostate health, so getting enough of the right nutrients is vital.

The prostate is a male gland that lies just beneath the bladder, wrapped around the urinary tube (urethra). From around the mid-forties onwards, the number of cells in the prostate often increases and the gland starts to enlarge. This is known as benign prostatic hyperplasia (BPH). The size and shape of a large chestnut during your twenties, the prostate more closely resembles a plump apricot by your forties, and can reach the size of a lemon by your sixties (occasionally enlarging to the size of a grapefruit, though this is uncommon). By the age of eighty, four out of five men have evidence of prostate enlargement, although only half go on to develop problematic symptoms.

Enlargement is thought to be a response to a changing balance between levels of testosterone, dihydrotestosterone and oestrogen hormones with age. As the prostate enlarges, it squeezes the urethra (which runs through its central lobe) to cause a variety of lower urinary tract symptoms, including:

- having to rush to the toilet to pass water
- passing water more frequently
- getting up at night to pass water
- straining to pass water
- a weak urinary stream
- starting and stopping mid-flow
- dribbling
- a sensation of not emptying the bladder fully
- urinary discomfort

## Prostate-health checklist

- **Maintain a healthy weight:** men with a waist circumference of more than 109 cm (43 in) are twice as likely to complain of lower urinary tract symptoms than men with a healthy waist size, and 38 per cent more likely to undergo surgery for BPH.
- **Take regular walks:** men who walk for two to three hours per week are 25 per cent less likely to develop troublesome BPH than those who don't.
- **Enjoy alcohol in moderation:** studies have found that men who consume three alcoholic drinks per day are half as likely to develop BPH as those who abstain, as alcohol reduces the effects of testosterone hormone.

## What causes it? PROSTATE ENLARGEMENT IS LINKED WITH:
- age • family history • obesity • high-fat diet • inactivity • type 2 diabetes
- high blood pressure

## Caution

If you develop lower urinary tract symptoms, seek medical advice to rule out prostate cancer as a possible cause. (NOTE: Having BPH does not increase your risk of having prostate cancer.)

## Foods that can help

- **Try following a low-fat, plant-based diet,** as this appears to be protective. Men who follow a traditional Japanese or Chinese diet (*see* overleaf) are less likely to develop symptoms of BPH than those following a Western diet, and they typically have a smaller prostate gland.
- **Eat plenty of fibre,** as this binds male hormones flushed out through the bile into the gut, so that less are reabsorbed. Sources include wholegrains, wholewheat bread and pasta, beans, fruit and vegetables, as well as the Japanese diet outlined overleaf.
- **Increase intake of zinc:** zinc is actively concentrated in prostate tissues and helps control its sensitivity to hormones. Zinc-rich foods include seafood (especially

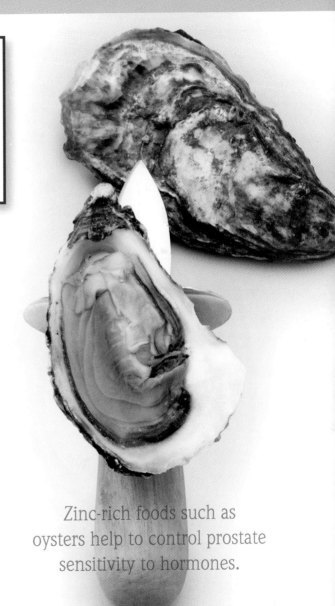

Zinc-rich foods such as oysters help to control prostate sensitivity to hormones.

oysters), wholegrains, bran, garlic, pumpkin seeds and pulses.

- **Consume more nuts and seeds**, as these contain essential fatty acids needed to make prostaglandins – hormone-like substances that are beneficial for prostate health (pumpkin seeds have long been traditionally used for prostate problems). They are also a good source of fibre.
- **Eat more tomatoes and tomato-based foods**, which have a high content of lycopene (a red carotenoid pigment). Men with the highest lycopene levels have been found to be up to 60 per cent less likely to develop prostate cancer than those with the lowest blood levels, suggesting it is beneficial for prostate health. Cooked tomatoes (ketchup, tomato sauces) provide the highest amounts.

## THE JAPANESE RECIPE FOR HEALTH

The traditional Japanese diet is low in fat (especially saturated fat), and consists of rice, soy products (such as soybeans, soymeal, tofu) and fish, together with legumes, grains and cruciferous plants (which include exotic members of the cabbage and turnip families, such as pak choi, kohlrabi and Chinese leaves). The diet is abundant in weak plant hormones (phytoestrogens such as isoflavones) that are converted into biologically active hormone-like substances by probiotic intestinal bacteria.

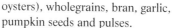

*Eat cruciferous plants such as pak choi.*

> ## DID YOU KNOW?
>
> The prostate produces secretions that nourish sperm, and acts like a valve to close off the bladder during ejaculation.

Studies comparing blood levels of phytoestrogens in Japanese and Finnish males found that Japanese levels were up to 110 times higher. These weak hormones are sufficiently similar to human oestrogens to trigger the production of a protein (sex hormone binding globulin) that mops up excess testosterone and reduces its effect on the prostate gland.

## Foods to avoid

A high-fat diet increases the risk of BPH. Studies show that men with high intakes of beef products are 25 per cent more likely to develop BPH than those with low intakes. High intakes of omega-6 fats (such as sunflower and corn oil) also increases the risk by 17 per cent, compared to men with low intakes. This is most likely because certain fatty acids act as building blocks for making androgen sex hormones.

## USEFUL SUPPLEMENTS

- **Zinc** helps to regulate prostate sensitivity to hormones
- **Lycopene** has a protective effect on prostate cell division
- **Soy isoflavones** have been linked with improved prostate health
- **Probiotic supplements** boost the conversion of dietary isoflavones to a more active form called equol
- **Saw palmetto** may reduce conversion of testosterone to the stronger dihydrotestosterone, helping the central part of an enlarged gland to shrink, and reducing the need to pass urine at night
- **Stinging nettle roots** contain beta-sitosterol and a variety of other sterols, and are often used together with saw palmetto
- **Reishi** has anti-androgen activity and can help to reduce male lower urinary tract symptoms
- **Evening primrose oil** contains essential fatty acids that are beneficial to prostate health

## Tomato & Pumpkin Seed Pesto

200 g (7 oz) pumpkin seeds
2 tbsp pumpkin seed oil
2 tbsp olive oil
2 cloves garlic
zest and juice of 1 unwaxed lemon

handful of fresh basil leaves
handful of sun-dried tomatoes
freshly ground black pepper

(serves 4)

- Place all the ingredients in a food processor and blend to your preferred pesto consistency. Season to taste with black pepper.
- Serve with wholewheat pasta, or spread on slices of fresh tomato to make canapés.

# Raynaud's disease

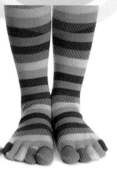

**Raynaud's affects an estimated** one in fifteen people, of whom two out of three are female. Eating foods that have a beneficial effect on the circulation can help – so reach for the garlic and improve your blood flow!

Raynaud's is a condition in which small arteries in the fingers and toes are overly sensitive to cold. They respond by constricting, so blood flow is severely reduced. As a result, digits turn white, with tingling or numbness. As a sluggish blood flow returns, the digits go blue and then turn bright red, with pain and unpleasant burning sensations. Most cases have no obvious cause initially. When associated with other specific diseases, such as scleroderma, it is known as Raynaud's phenomenon.

In one study of sixty-four people with Raynaud's disease, half went on to develop a connective tissue disorder, such as scleroderma (an autoimmune condition in which antibodies attack tissues to cause skin thickening) over the following eight years.

## Foods that can help

- **Go for garlic!** Garlic has a beneficial effect on blood vessel dilation and blood stickiness, helping to improve circulation through small arteries and veins. Studies show it dilates arterioles

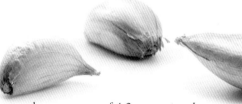

by an average of 4.2 per cent and venules by 5.9 per cent, improving blood flow to the skin and nail folds by as much as 50 per cent. Platelet clumping is significantly decreased after a dose equivalent to half a clove and lasts for three hours; some of the ingredients in garlic appear to be as potent as aspirin in this respect.
- **Eat more oily fish,** such as salmon, mackerel or herring; this helps to reduce blood stickiness and

## Raynaud's checklist

- **Keep hands and feet as warm as possible.**
- **Stop smoking,** as this further constricts small arteries.
- **Avoid sudden or extreme changes in temperature.**

## What causes it? RAYNAUD'S DISEASE IS LINKED WITH:

• family history • using vibrating power tools • arterial diseases (such as atherosclerosis, blood clotting disorders) • connective tissue diseases (for example, rheumatoid arthritis, scleroderma, SLE) • some prescribed drugs (such as beta-blockers)

can improve circulation to the peripheries (*see also* page 28).

• **Eat ginger,** which has a natural warming effect.
• **Increase intake of magnesium,** found in beans, nuts, wholegrains, seafood and dark green leafy vegetables, as this has beneficial effects on the circulation.

### USEFUL SUPPLEMENTS

• **Gingko biloba extracts** and **omega-3 fish oils** can improve blood flow to the peripheries
• **Vitamin E supplements** are often helpful, as their antioxidant action helps to reduce spasm of small blood vessels

 **Salmon with Ginger-lime Aioli**

4 salmon steaks

**For the aioli:**
3 tbsp low-fat mayonnaise
3 tbsp low-fat crème fraîche
3 cloves garlic, crushed

thumb-sized piece of fresh ginger, grated
zest and juice of 1 lime
freshly ground black pepper

(serves 4)

• To make the aioli, combine all of the ingredients except the salmon, and mix well. Season to taste, then cover and refrigerate for 30 minutes.
• Meanwhile, preheat the grill to a medium heat and lightly grill the salmon steaks until the flesh is just set. Serve with the aioli.

Oily fish can improve circulation.

# FURMER READING *Other recommended titles by Dr Sarah Brewer*

*Nutrition: A Beginner's Guide*, Oneworld, 2013

*Live Longer Look Younger*, Connections Book Publishing, 2012

*Death: A Survival Guide*, Quercus, 2011

*Cut Your Stress*, Quercus, 2010

*Essential Guide to Vitamins, Minerals and Herbal Supplements*, Right Way, 2010

*The Human Body*, Quercus, 2009

*Cut Your Cholesterol*, Quercus, 2009

*Low-Cholesterol Cookbook for Dummies*, Wiley, 2009

*Natural Health Guru: Overcoming Arthritis*, Duncan Baird, 2009

*Natural Health Guru: Overcoming Asthma*, Duncan Baird, 2009

*Natural Health Guru: Overcoming High Blood Pressure*, Duncan Baird, 2008

*Natural Health Guru: Overcoming Diabetes*, Duncan Baird, 2008

*Menopause for Dummies*, Wiley, 2007

*Thyroid for Dummies*, Wiley, 2006

*Arthritis for Dummies*, Wiley, 2006

*Natural Approaches to Diabetes*, Piatkus, 2005

*Intimate Relations: Living and Loving in Later Life*, Age Concern, 2004

*The Total Detox Plan*, Carlton, 2000, 2011

# INDEX

## PICTURE CREDITS
**Cover** iStockphoto/Thinkstock
Recipe panel (repeats throughout): dowilukas/iStockphoto
Cooking pot logo (repeats throughout): iStockphoto/Thinkstock

**iStockphoto** 21

**ShutterStockphoto,Inc** annata78 130; antos777 108; Ake Avalanchez 38; BestPhotoStudio 2–3; Nikita Chisnikov 51; Steven Collins 151; daffodilred 87; Dionisvera 157; eurobanks 39; Fenton 166; Food photography 58; foodonwhite 138; Foodpictures 65; Goodluz 140; Oliver Hoffman 139; Julia Ivantsova 34; jannoon028 6–7; Mark LaMoyne 86; Christine Langer-Pueschel 66r; MidoSemsem 143; Sergey Mironov 42–3; Monkey Business Images 128; motorolka 64; nanka 142; Pefkos 77b; Richard Peterson 109; Anette Linnea Rasmussen 161; rolfik 159; Zdenek Rosenthaler 119; Elena Schweitzer 141; topseller 35, 78r; Suzanne Tucker 62l; VictoriaKh 77t; voranat 107; wavebreakmedia 30–31; WimL 149; withGod 57; Peter Zijistra 131, 133

**Thinkstock** BananaStock 52, 82, 132; Brand X Pictures 84; Comstock 112; Creatas 129; Digital vision 32, 69, 72–3, 89, 100, 154b, 168; Dorling Kindersley RF 95; F1online 167; Fuse 8–9, 49, 114; Hemera 16, 22, 74t, 122, 134, 156, 164; iStockphoto 5, 10, 10–11, 12, 15, 17, 18, 19, 20, 23, 24, 25, 26, 27, 28, 29, 33, 36t, 36b, 37, 40b, 43, 44, 45, 46, 48, 50, 52–3, 54, 56, 59, 60, 61, 62r, 66l, 66–7, 68, 71, 74b, 76, 78l, 79, 80, 81, 83, 85, 88, 90, 91, 93, 94, 96, 97, 98, 99, 103, 104, 105, 106, 110, 111, 113, 115, 116t, 116b, 117, 118, 120, 121, 123, 124t, 124b, 125, 126, 127, 135, 136, 137, 144, 145, 146, 147, 148, 152, 153, 154t, 155, 158, 160, 162, 163, 165, 169, 170l, 171; Polka Dot 70b, 72; Purestock 102; Stockbyte 14, 40t, 92, 150; Top Photo Group 13, 170r; Wavebreak Media 70t

## ACKNOWLEDGEMENTS
I would like to thank everyone who has been so helpful in providing research papers and information for the insights explored in this book.

### EDDISON•SADD EDITIONS
**Creative Director** Nick Eddison
**Managing Editor** Tessa Monina
**Proofreader** Nicola Hodgson
**Indexer** Marie Lorimer
**Designer** Jane McKenna
**Picture research administration** Rosie Taylor
**Production** Sarah Rooney